HUMAN PSYCHOLOGY AS SEEN THROUGH THE DREAM

Founded by C. K. Ogden

The International Library of Psychology

GENERAL PSYCHOLOGY
In 38 Volumes

HUMAN PSYCHOLOGY AS SEEN THROUGH THE DREAM

JULIA TURNER

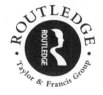

First published in 1924 by
Kegan Paul, Trench, Trubner & Co., Ltd.

Reprinted 1999, 2000 by
Routledge
2 Park Square, Milton Park, Abingdon, Oxfordshire OX14 4RN
711 Third Avenue, New York, NY 10017

First issued in paperback 2014

Routledge is an imprint of the Taylor and Francis Group, an informa company

Transferred to Digital Printing 2006

© 1924 Julia Turner

British Library Cataloguing in Publication Data
A CIP catalogue record for this book
is available from the British Library

Human Psychology as Seen Through the Dream
ISBN 978-0-415-21046-1 (hbk)
ISBN 978-0-415-75811-6 (pbk)

General Psychology: 38 Volumes
ISBN 978-0-415-21129-1
The International Library of Psychology: 204 Volumes
ISBN 978-0-415-19132-6

Truth is within ourselves ; it takes no rise
From outward things, whate'er you may believe.
There is an inmost centre in us all,
Where truth abides in fulness ; and around,
Wall upon wall, the gross flesh hems it in,
This perfect clear perception—which is truth.
A baffling and perverting carnal mesh
Blinds it, and makes all error : and to *KNOW*
Rather consists in opening out a way
Whence the imprisoned splendour may escape,
Than in effecting entry for a light
Supposed to be without.

.   .   .   .
                    See this soul of ours !
How it strives weakly in the child, is loosed
In manhood, clogged by sickness, back compelled
By age and waste, set free at last by death :
Why is it, flesh enthralls it or enthrones ?
What is this flesh we have to penetrate ?

.   .   .   .
                    One man shall crawl
Through life surrounded with all stirring things,
Unmoved ; and he goes mad : and from the wreck
Of what he was, by his wild talk alone,
You first collect how great a spirit he hid.
Therefore, set free the soul alike in all,
Discovering the true laws by which the flesh
Accloys the spirit !

                              Paracelsus, Bk. I.
                              ROBERT BROWNING.

PREFACE

THE present book is an attempt to supplement the slight sketch of the Anxiety Hypothesis put forward in *The Psychology of Self-Consciousness*. The former book aimed at explaining the difference between the perceptual and conceptual aspects of life, and at showing, by reference to general literature, the anxiety elements in human thought. In the present book in Part I anxiety is described as arising through the reciprocal actions of *introjection* and *projection* to supply the warp and woof not only of individual character, but of an unseen spiritual self ; in Part II is traced out the sinouus course of the dream life conceived as a dramatic cycle.

The value of introspection on the Anxiety Hypothesis is frankly advocated, not only in particular as a therapeutic method, but also as an educational method of high value. Every reflecting being must introspect ; there is a methodical introspection which is valuable, whereas unmethodical introspection is difficult and sometimes injurious.

Thanks are due to Messrs. Burns, Oates and Washbourne ; Longmans, Green and Co. ; Macmillan and Co. ; Methuen and Co. ; John Watkins ; T. Fisher Unwin ; for permission to use material quoted from books published by them.

AN ANSWER TO SOME CRITICISMS OF THE ANXIETY HYPOTHESIS.

I gather that I have failed to make entirely clear my position in regard to two points which affect dream interpretation. Both affect the exact nature of the ultimate conflict in the subliminal sphere.

1. The conflict in the unconscious is *not*, on the Anxiety Hypothesis, between the perceptual and the conceptual. It is, on the contrary, wholly conceptual. It is the titanic struggle from which all anxiety experience for the rest of existence derives both its terrors and its sublimity. In the ultimate conflict the perceptual is *always only symbol*. But in the pseudo-unconscious there must be frequent conflicts between the conceptual and perceptual interests. This phase, like that of the phantasy life with which it is commonly associated, may lead to a veritable forty years of wandering in the wilderness. There is plenty of material forthcoming reflecting the struggle in which the perceptual, as such, tempts the unwary conceptual subject (a) *from myth*, the stories of Pan, the Satyrs, Centaurs, imprisonment in trees ; (b) *from dreams*, uncouth monsters, and dreams in which the clothing of the upper part of the body (coat or bodice) is not in keeping with that of the lower part of the body (trousers or skirt) ; (c) *from child psychology*, the child's representations of animals and man, the latter particularly, with very little body part. This conflict is a problem of projection ; it affects the educationist very particularly. Difficulties in negotiating this phase are among the evil effects of the child's language insufficiency and of the limitations of sympathy and even of knowledge in the human race in its functions as guardians of its youth. It explains the application of the word *dirty* to satisfaction of the instincts, an attitude to the matter which the dream mind supports in referring to displaced energy.

2. Not less is it incorrect, in my opinion, to say that the conflict of the dream is between *the ego-impulse and sexuality*. The very use of these terms shows that the critic is still thinking of the conceptual faculties of the human mind rather as a sublimation of instinct than as a new creation, as the Anxiety Hypothesis conceives it. To call the instinct of self-preservation the *ego-impulse* does not alter the fact that what is under discussion is *instinct*. Both the instinct of race-preservation (sexuality) and the instinct of self-preservation (ego-impulse) lend themselves as symbolism and *both work both ways*. Some forms of sexual pre-occupation are the symbol of death unto life, some of death unto death. Some substances eaten (knowledge and experience " taken in ") are nutritious ; some deleterious ; some even poisonous. All physiological function symbolises psychic function and it may subserve either selfishness or self-surrender. This is the heart of the symbolism, involving a choice which is the central fact. Even when expressed as a love romance the concern of the nuclear conflict of the dream is the surrender of life to Him Who gave it.

The deepest concern of the inner life, as known to us through the dream, seems to be the training of the will to re-enact with open vision, in relation to an unseen Source of Life, the infant's original surrender to the mother after the agitation of the initial sparking situation or situations. This concern is ultimately one belonging to the conceptual sphere.

Professor Freud, in his latest work, is arriving at the idea of a second determinant principle. He calls it death. He misses the conceptual subtleties in regard to it, as he formerly did in relation to sexuality. Professor Freud's work has opened one door—an outer door—but it is only when a symbolic value is given to his ultimates that the inner door of the temple of Psyche can be opened.

CONTENTS

PART I

THE DREAM IS THE PSYCHOLOGICAL APPARATUS FOR HARMONISING EXPERIENCE

PART II

THE ANXIETY DRAMA

xi

HUMAN PSYCHOLOGY
AS SEEN THROUGH THE DREAM

PART I

THE DREAM IS THE PSYCHOLOGICAL
APPARATUS HARMONISING EXPERIENCE

CHAPTER I

INTRODUCTION

What's Hecuba to him or he to Hecuba ?
(Hamlet)

HAMLET has been interviewing the Players. The sight of them had recalled the fact that when last entertained by this troupe the leader had declaimed a scene from the final act in a play on the siege of Troy. Hamlet asks to hear it again. The passage describes the slaying of Priam and the pitiful plight of his aged queen, bereaved of husband, sons and daughters, fleeing from her desolated home :—

> " Barefoot up and down, threatening the flames
> With bisson rheum ; a clout upon that head
> Where late the diadem stood ; and, for a robe,
> About her lank and all o'er teemèd loins,
> A blanket, in the alarum of fear caught up."

The piece had never been acted; it was "caviare to the general," but in the recitation the Player had expressed signs of emotion, all his own.

Now Hamlet is alone. The Players have received the Prince's commands and for a moment the bitter frenzy of Hamlet's own anxiety is mingled with a fellow feeling for the man whose voice had trembled and eyes become suffused with tears, as he pronounced phrase by phrase the description of the sufferings of Hecuba.

What's Hecuba to him or he to Hecuba?

Hecuba is for the moment everything to the player who enters *sympathetically* into the telling of her pathetic story. That is to say, for the purposes of his own anxiety life he "identifies himself with," or feels himself one with, Hecuba; her desolated condition is for him a picture or image of his own inner life. For Hamlet himself this is no less true. We remember that it is Hamlet who asks to have the poem recited. On the occasion when he originally heard it some inner impulse must have appropriated the mimic situation, some intuition in him having singled out the fate of Priam and Hecuba amid the ruins of Troy as *prefigurative* of his own destiny.

It is in virtue of our capacity for identifying ourselves with others that a theatrical representation affords us interest, and there is, moreover, a selective principle at work in the process which brings it about that the obvious parallel in the representation is not by any means necessarily the character which appeals most to any given spectator at any given time. What two beings could seem more remote than a man in his prime and the aged Hecuba in flight? Well might Hamlet ask, " What's Hecuba to him or he to Hecuba ? " And if Hamlet is surprised at the actor, the surprise applies in his case even more. One might have expected that the son and heir of a king, at the period of life that Hamlet was, having just completed his studies and returned to his father's state, would find his interest centre, not in the stricken consort of the unsuccessful defender of Troy, but in the triumphant besieger insinuating his troops into the city by the ruse of the Great Wooden Horse.

On the principle of identification, we find people in daily life expressing sympathy with children in distress or with animals in suffering; we might even go further and say that, at least in part, our regret over a broken ornament or defaced book is derived from the same source, namely, identification of the self with the object on which our feeling expends itself. Without a doubt, the other side of the picture holds equally. We are as capable of identifying ourselves with the successful hero. Which type of object shall claim the larger amount of interest will depend upon our mood, but the identification process is at work in both cases. Projection is a word highly applicable to this identification process, for it implies that there is an interior source furnishing the image of the self which corresponds with the external object capable of arresting the subject's attention. This interior

source is the " Anxiety Drama " of the dream
life.

In Part II of this book I shall attempt to describe
and explain the Anxiety Drama in more detail.   In
the *Psychology of Self-Consciousness* I have
shown that it originates in the sensory images
derived, in the period of sensori-motor inco-ordination and language-inadequacy of babyhood, from
emotional situations in which the child is directly
or indirectly concerned.   At this stage of his conceptual life the subject is alone, and the sensory
images are confused with emotional states which
the originals of the picture aroused in himself.   In
group-subjects, the same emotion is *induced* in the
" patient " as the latter sees expressed by the
" agent " in the situation; an image of the
mother's angry or pleased face is the immediate
reflection of his own emotion.   Henceforward that
image is capable of being revived together with the
associated emotion.   In the waking life, with the
acquisition of language, the image habit tends to
lapse for ordinary purposes, and energy escapes
along speech and motor paths.   In the waking
mental process known as imagination, mental pictures continue to find a place, but they have less
vividness and are subject to control; in the dream,
the older habit persists in its original guise, the
images, however, being constantly replenished
from current experience.   That this replenishing
process goes on in us unobserved is shown by the
fact that dreams reproduce elements of experience
which, at the time the experience took place, did

not, so far as we can see, particularly impress us. This process may be called Introjection.

The image or symbol habit is created and carried on for the purpose of an inner life which I have called the conceptual or self-conscious life. It is a life detached from the actual pleasures and pains of material existence. Over against this life lies the life of the flesh, the ordinary animal existence —the perceptual life, as I have called it in the *Psychology of Self-Consciousness*—the heritage of man as a species, the highest species which has appeared in the evolutionary series. Perceptual life is concerned with the interests of the organism. To bring the Conceptual and Perceptual into relationship is the function of the Anxiety phase of self-consciousness, revealing itself normally in the dream and in phantasy. Anxiety is wakened in infancy, probably with abruptness, and possibly in a situation which involves pain for the subject. I have called the process the " sparking," using the analogy of the starting of a petrol motor.

The above division of the mental life into conceptual, perceptual and anxiety experience includes every vital phenomenon known to the human subject. It excludes neither the lowest animal function, on the one hand, nor the most ideal aspiration on the other; it includes the normal and the so-called abnormal. The theory which regards the higher impulses of our nature as something *extra*, something imported from outside, is one which I fail to find confirmed in the dream. The *de novo* theory assumes that mankind has some private

B

source of knowledge, an idea which seems strange when looked at more closely, for everything in the subjective world, the world of sensation, feeling and thought, must surely proceed from the one source, the Life-Principle itself. That pros and cons are bandied between opposite parties in the discussion of all the most important human concerns—especially in the discussion of the most arresting problem with which the human mind can deal, that of personal immortality—merely illustrates the fact that development of anxiety proceeds along two opposite lines, following conceptual and perceptual experience respectively. Every anxiety phenomenon illustrates this bifurcation of interest, one line following the course of experience which recedes into an inner source, the other the course of interest which flows out into the phenomenal environment.

The inner life unfolds for waking consciousness as the result of " Introjecting " the happenings encountered in the material world; on the other hand life lived among one's human fellows is regulated, if not enhanced, by the projection on to it of something supplied from within which gives form and continuity and purpose to the life of self-consciousness. To bring the two aspects of life into a single act of mental vision is the highest human accomplishment. To achieve this would be to turn all phenomenal functions into a sacrament —to spiritualise every experience of sense.

This is in effect the meaning of the saying of Jesus, " If thine eye be single thy whole body shall be full of light.'' The eye referred to is obviously not the physical eye, but the focus of the Life-Principle become self-conscious in the human being. To include in a single sweep of vision both the life of material things and the life of spiritual things is to have the body full of light; to see only the things of sense is to have the light that is within become darkness for waking experience.

The object of this treatise is to describe how human life develops conceptually. Part I deals with the reciprocal processes of Introjection and Projection; in Part II I endeavour to show how the study of the dream may be used to serve the purpose of unification of experience.

Through the study of the dream it becomes apparent by what mechanism it happens that the whole world enters the soul of man, there to create out of animal emotions a new and higher fact—a thought life. The infant is a creature of massive feeling, in quality negative and positive, feeling associated, at this stage, as in his immediate animal ancestors, with the instincts. After the sparking the child associates his feelings mainly with the personalities, human and animal, in his environment; a slow laborious process at first, it grows with exercise. The first situations arouse pleasure and displeasure in gross; habituation induces more measured reaction. Feelings have become the personalities among which they (the feelings) are distributed. As experience enlarges, the '' dream population '' grows and develops and the scope of their activities enlarges, with the result that the

child's feelings, erstwhile massive and simply negative or positive, become widely distributed, what
they stand for more widely discriminated and their
content less feeling than thought. At first just
" good " or " bad," (*i.e.*, fearful or pleasurable in
relation to sensory criteria), the dream personalities
become good or bad in varying degrees in relation
to other experience which gives knowledge to the
child of the laws of his own being. Through a
special class of dream, of which the " falling "
dream is typical, the child learns subconsciously
that the law of his life is that the vital energy should
rise in his nervous apparatus. The " fall " dream
is not the fall of the subject but of the vital energy
in the nervous system. [1]

The dream warns the child what he should really
fear because it breaks the law of his own being.
As he learns to choose good and avoid evil, or *vice
versa,* character develops. The images importing
that which is most feared, whether good or evil—
for both are or may be feared—are banished and
become forgotten, " dissociated," a very apt
technical word. The dreams of infantile origin
show fear of that which will break the law and pre-
cipitate consequences foreboding danger, and on
the other hand they make into a thing of beauty, or
at least a thing to be desired, that which is in
accordance with the laws of vital energy. All is at
first referred only within and all hangs together,
producing the effect of a dramatic representation.

[1] These psycho-physical problems cannot be adequately dealt
with at this stage. See Appendix I, No. 1.

This is a process which forges thought out of feeling and is perpetually tempering the instrument and sharpening its edge. Finer and finer differences between these feeling-saturated thoughts are perpetually coming to light in the child's experience, the relations of each to the other and each to the whole becoming clearer. These are the thought relations as ordinarily understood (the logical relations). Projection is the process by which the correspondences between the interior and exterior worlds are re-established or sought to be re-established. It is a process which is subject to many difficulties.

The dream, we may assume, is only part of the whole mechanism of mind organisation, a process which will be going on in ordinary circumstances as steadily as the metabolism of the physical body, with which, indeed, the dream compares it. In the dream normally the subject's immediate experiences are staged in order that he may see whither his line of present-day experience is leading and how it is related to the whole. The " fearful " in the dream, far from attaching to physical and external values, is really directed to keeping intact a higher self and providing for the expansion of spiritual energies. By projection, the subject re-discovers in the external universe the creations of his interior life and applies them to it. Hence the rational mind as we contact it embodies the thought relations which have developed between the various parts of the dream life. Because the invariable nucleus of the dream symbolism brings into relation the body and the

" unseen self," the bulk of the thought life of mankind is essentially the same. Again, because all other symbolism is highly flexible, involving as it does individual and racial differences, the thought of every human soul shows marked variations.

CHAPTER II

THE INAUGURATION OF INTROJECTION AND PROJECTION

A spark disturbs our clod.
(*Rabbi ben Ezra*, R. Browning)

THE medium of exchange between experience of the inner life and experience as we understand it in a phenomenal environment is in the first instance symbolism. A symbol is something concrete, something familiar to sense, which is adopted to represent experience of the inner life. Practically everything which the human mind can take cognisance of, is capable, by furnishing symbolism, of assisting towards the harmonisation of experience.

I will attempt to trace what appears to me to be the probable course of the rise of the symbol habit in the individual.

The baby, at first merely an animal subject, has self-consciousness " sparked " in him in some situation involving intense emotion. The situation is in all likelihood one in which the child's guardian counters his will in a quite unmistakable fashion. The change of countenance, the signs of displeasure, in a face which has hitherto looked into his with nothing but gentleness and love, provide a momentous experience; the significance is heightened if infliction of pain accompanies the essential signs of displeasure. It arouses a mixed feeling of fear and hate.

As the perceptual subject quickens in the mother's womb, so the conceptual subject is quickened when the baby subject first reads displeasure in her face.

Because in the helpless subject fear cannot. activate the flight-impulse—*i.e.*, the subject cannot run away—his reactions mark a new departure in the mental life. [1] We may assume that the sensory image becomes endowed with superior vividness and with permanence. The angry face, the raised voice, any significant movement made by the object he confronts and all somatic accompaniments of his own, will henceforward tend to associate themselves with any future situation in which the subject cannot so react as to secure immediate safety, *i.e.*, with every anxiety situation. Henceforth the image embodies the particular emotion. It exists for the sake of the emotion, and whenever the emotion recurs, the image, we may suppose, will at the same time be revived in memory. Again, the smiling face, which succeeds the angry one, expressing forgiveness and a renewal of the love relation, is on the same principle assimilated for pleasurable experience. There follow before long images of other angry and pleased faces; for the same emotions as expressed by every individual must present differences, since no two persons are affected in quite the same fashion, and their capacity for instilling fear or suggesting well-being will

[1] I have heard it argued that the child's tears, cries and aimless contortions may carry off the energy generated, but I contend that nothing short of *flight* can really satisfy the animal under the influence of fear.

likewise vary. The father's mode of expressing anger and pleasure will be different from the mother's, and these will both differ from the expression of the same emotions as seen in the face of each one of all the members of the baby's little group; yet the facial image of anger in all will bear a certain resemblance and so also will the facial image of happy pleasedness. Consequently, whenever the infant suffers because he desires to alleviate his condition and cannot—if only because he cannot reach an object or effect any other change in his circumstances which would remove an inconvenience or produce positive satisfaction—the symbolic face will present itself on the field of memory as it does in the dreams of the adult. The same thing will happen in respect to auditory images. In both cases, it will be the *prepotent* stimulus which will survive, *i.e.*, the face of the person who instils most fear, or the voice expressing for the little subject the most alluring sense of pleasure, will secure priority, a quality in a stimulus which in psychology is expressed by the word *prepotency*.

As the self-conscious habit becomes fixed, images corresponding to emotions slightly different in quality from the above will add themselves to the picture gallery. Situations in which the child sees anger directed against another child will impress on the awakening self-consciousness an image of fear as expressed by the threatened child. It is not necessarily the face which provides the image, it may be the part threatened, *e.g.*, a subject remembers seeing the button of a sister's frock flicked from

the back with a stick by the father. The visual image
chronicles just the objects involved, back, button
and stick. This is an entirely different experience
from that provided by a situation in which the child
himself is blamed directly, and so, also, is the
picture of the little culprit's reactions of tearful
repentance different from the vision which presents
itself to the subject when his own reinstatement is in
question. The little brother or sister who provokes
jealousy or resentment, the image of suffering
expressed by another child with an injury to hand
or knee, all, as memory pictures, become associated
with the feelings that are seeking expression. All
such sensory images become vehicles of emotional
states. Attempts are early made by the guardians
to teach the child to name (a) objects; *e.g.*, father,
mother, pussy, food, and also (b) the moral and
aesthetic qualities of such objects, *e.g.*, good and
naughty, of pussy; clean and dirty, of hands, face,
etc.; but it would be too soon to attempt to provide names for anything not *concrete*. Where,
therefore, the appropriate describing of states of
mind is concerned the impressions are conveyed
by facial distortions. Thus, a dirty or disagreeable
thing evokes a pantomimic expression of disgust in
the face of the guardian.

Bodily attitudes, in fine, provide the first symbols.
Their function is to convey emotional values.
In the dream, the bodies of people and parts of the
body represent emotions and emotional attitudes.
This is the class of symbols first elaborated and it
has in every way a determining effect on the whole
habit of symbolisation.

The entire process by which experience is appropriated for the inner life under the symbolising habit is called in this treatise Introjection. I have suggested in the *Psychology of Self-Consciousness* that Introjection is allied to Passive Sympathy. The whole subject, however, requires the most careful investigation. Images assimilated by the self-conscious subject to express emotion represent, it must be remembered, *the subject's own states of mind.* All images in the dream are, therefore, to be interpreted subjectively. There are no people in the dream, strictly speaking, but only sensory images embodying the mental states of the dreamer.

This is so because the dream is a survival from the first stage of self-consciousness, a period when the subject is unable to distinguish, in conceptual experience, between the I and the Not-I.

While self-consciousness is dawning, Introjection must proceed apace. As there are few ways in which the child's energy can flow off in reaction, introjected material must accumulate. So soon as the motor paths are open, the reciprocal process of Projection will begin. The child's first efforts at Projection are characteristic; he now takes some trivial object he can handle freely, such as a doll or other toy, and manipulates it for the purpose of expressing anxiety situations. For dawning self-consciousness the object is the *self.* In proportion to his vivacity the child will throw himself more or less energetically into his play; he will croon over the toy and expend affection on it as his mother has on him; in a little while he will push or throw it away, actions again reminiscent of situations in which he has suffered " rejection." The toy is always fetched back and the double process repeated. A vast amount of curiosity accompanies the experimentation. The toy is turned over and over and minutely examined, outside certainly, and inside if possible. Later on, but probably in some cases only, there is exhibitionism too. The exhibitionistic little actor will insist that interest shall be taken in him while he is engaged in his play.

Introjection and Projection are obviously reciprocal processes at this stage. A little child has no sooner sufficiently mastered the meaning of a situation than he proceeds to reproduce it in mimic representation. It is significant that mock anxiety at this stage and all through life shares in common with serious dramatic art the description " play."

It is not considered advisable that a child be allowed to linger too long at this stage of spontaneous representation of anxiety situations. It is too valuable a period to be lost, and, provided he is taught by way of play, education cannot take over too early the direction of the Introjection and Projection habits. Otherwise, the subject may become too introspective, or, if he is of a lively disposition, curiosity will prompt the introjection of undesirable situations.

The process of education cannot with safety neglect to observe that the balance be kept between the rights of the inner subjective life and the interests of the material world, for the harmonisation of which the processes of Introjection and Projection exist.   It must be remembered that at this early stage, very particularly, introjected experience furnishes the apparatus through which the ultimate values of Life-as-a-whole are capable of expressing themselves.   Here is the cradle of art and of originality, indeed, of genuine individuality.   It is necessary that provision be made for ensuring that the inner life shall have *depth,* as well as the outer life *extent* of interest.   Time-honoured channels for furnishing the inner man with appropriate pabulum are religion, music, colour and nature from every aspect.   The great importance of the period of life which sees anxiety inaugurated has been well brought out by Professor Freud, but I doubt if justice has been fully done to it and whether its *true* importance has been made clear.

This is the period for the defining of the relations of the I and the Not-I ; the organ of knowledge is the superficies of the body, together with the alimentary tract, which is biologically continuous with the external surface of the body.   Both are the seat of the most exquisite pleasure and pain and it is a picture of tactile sensation and metabolic change which is created by experience of this period.   In respect to the life of the senses, much that is naturally pleasurable is repressed in the child, and at the same time much artificial suffering is imposed on him.   On the one hand, the child is denied the freedom of his own person ; on the other, his tender little body is clothed in garments which, at best, restrict his activities ; again, his diet is regulated and nauseous physic prescribed ; occasionally bodily

punishment is meted out to him. His bodily superficies and alimentary tract are, in fact, the meeting-
ground of the I and the Not-I ; anxiety results and
an atonement has to be made. So important a
symbol in the dream is nutrition that it is doubtful
whether it may not contain the original mystery of
communion between the self and the Ruling
Powers. Hunger and pain first initiate us into the
secrets of life and death. All appetite, the seeking
of positive satisfaction, is the *call of life* expressed
through the apparatus of the organism ; pain the
bitter *plaint of life* in this same aspect, in its encounter with hostile agencies which are stronger than it
and against which it cannot maintain itself without
conflict. Hence hunger and pain become for the
self-conscious subject symbolic of his yearning for
the great source of life which is both within and
without him. Communion expresses the subject's
deep satisfaction with that life of which he and his
Deity partake in common, also the sense of his
dependence on the All-of-life and the need to remain
rooted therein. Religion may originally have been
the projected expression of those deepest unspoken
and unspeakable yearnings, and the earliest
religious ritual would consequently revolve round
nutrition as a symbol. Religion that was anterior
to the knowledge of the facts of impregnation would
be of this character.

Certainly, in many nervous conditions, the subject presents a picture of such sheer preoccupation
with safety as to seem to leave aside all the ordinary
sexual preoccupations on which dream psycholo-

gists lay so much stress.   The maturing of the reproductive system and knowledge of the obvious facts of sexuality brings with it a second stage both in the evolution of religion and in the evolution of individual self-consciousness.   Adolescence is a further development, a re-birth into self-consciousness.   The extreme type of anxiety subject seems never to have negotiated this new development; certainly life is rendered infinitely more complicated for the conceptual subject by the advent of the reproductive function.   Sexuality overlays the earlier metabolic symbolism with another symbol system, which in some respects shows correspondence with the earlier one, but which in other respects is new and startling, if not opposite in sense. It is inability to produce harmony as between these two symbol systems which is the special anxiety problem of adolescence.

CHAPTER III

INTROJECTION AND PROJECTION AND THEIR RELATION TO LANGUAGE

That rash humour which my mother gave me.

(Julius Cæsar)

BEFORE the child is able to communicate with those about him, his conceptual life is defined by a rapidly accumulating series of images, mainly visual, which tend to be revived and to coalesce with new ones whenever emotional situations arise.   With the above tendency, which is the passive aspect (Introjection), there coexists a conative tendency—a tendency to *create* dramatic situations which express past emotional situations (Projection).   The latter tendency represents the delayed motor reactions of the stimuli received during the period of motor inco-ordination; hence the play of childhood. When playing, everything that the child does with an object he can dominate is reminiscent of anxiety situations he has been in, situations which were favourable to him, and again, situations which were unfavourable to him, the object dominated being for the subject always the self.   There emerges the idea of being safe or saved, together with the opposite idea of being in a state where the subject is unsafe, or even " lost."   We may suppose that when the child is unhappy he will compensate himself by creating a situation suggestive of happiness, and when he is happy he may venture to create situations of the opposite character. The Projection phase also results from an immediate experience or " stimulus." In either case, when once the emotion is in train, there is a tendency to reproduce the whole of it. Anxiety once aroused may tend to discharge itself completely, e.g., a child in disgrace may tend to discharge all the emotional content of the complex situation or situations revived by the immediate experience. The violent anger he expresses, apparently directed against someone or something outside, really belongs to the cycle of his own subjective life. Further, from what we observe through the dream of the *law of balance,* we may suppose that the violence of anger will be succeeded by an emotional phase of the opposite character (repentance) the intensity of which will equal that of the first. We must believe that emotional differences in conceptual subjects are regulated, not by the immediate situation, but by situations previously introjected; certainly, anger reactions in a very little child are purely subjective, and, as projections, quite aimless. Unless fresh projections supervene early in life to soften unduly violent exhibitions of emotion, the latter will tend to become fixed as habits of mind, whether submerged or in the waking life. In other words, sympathetic training at this earliest period is of the utmost importance in forming character—character including the buried anxiety life as well as manifestations of anxiety in consciousness. Apart from any ques-

c

tion of physical heredity, the immediate guardians of the infant are in a very special sense responsible for what the child will tend to become as a conceptual subject. We are impressed, however, as dream psychologists, with the fact that, fortunately, not only is character most flexible, but that in the inner life of man the subject is ever striving for " salvation," *i.e.*, subjectively for internal unity, and, so far as he is rational, objectively for a place in the love of his fellows and in that of a Supreme Being.

Besides direct emotional training, opportunities for exploring the environment will assist indirectly in correcting reactions unduly charged with affect. A second class of objects which the infant encounters are those which he cannot dominate, either because he has not sufficient knowledge of the properties of minds and bodies or because he is not strong enough to overcome the opposition the latter offer—if it be only a question of the inertia of matter. His attention is arrested by the reaction of such objects evoked by his actions, or by the absence of reaction, and a fresh crop of introjected images result. The difference observed between his actions on these objects and their reactions will become finer and finer. As the introjected images multiply, each successive crop of mental images will provide more and more discriminative emotional variations until the emotion is practically eliminated, partly through sheer division, partly through shifting of attention on to the devices suggested by intelligence for overcoming opposition. [1] The tendency to eliminate emotion holds, except in exceptional cases, wherever the bare problem of dominance is involved. Where experience is accompanied by marked pain, as in contact with hard objects or with fire, the memory picture of such contact will not, of course, cease to have a strong emotional content, and the same will be true of objects which are capable of giving pleasure more particularly. All emotion attaching to objects in the conceptual life may be termed " symbolic efficacy." This is the " affect " of which dream psychologists write and of which they remark that it has a strong tendency to become displaced. It is ultimately derived, as the law of displacement put forward by these writers implies, from the earliest emotional situations in which self-consciousness is sparked, *i.e.,* from situations in which the earliest guardians of the child are the important factor.

The acquisition of language brings about certain very important changes. Language embodies all the achievements of the processes peculiar to the self-consciousness of generations and generations of ancestors. Every word is a symbol acquired originally through highly significant conceptual experience. The child at first acquires this symbol-system with difficulty, but as experience proceeds he rapidly enters more and more into its spirit. He seems to touch the *Weltgeist* here. With some subjects, the illumination which language brings

[1] This practical application of energy may appropriately be called *sublimation* in contradistinction to *transmutation* of energy a subconscious process with which sublimation of energy must not on any account be confounded.

expresses itself as intensity. We know people who repeat the same phrases and the same stories, which seem to bring more pleasure or fear with every repetition. Others again revel in an extent of language, and early acquire phrases which embody ideas derived from experience with which, as present-day subjects, they can have no intimacy, words, for instance, belonging to, at least for them, dead and gone " ologies," *e.g.*, mythologies and astrology, and as quickly acquire the language in which new ideas are presented. Since all human experience embodies the same problem of salvation presented in an endless variety of forms, universality of taste in language exhibits, I presume, a deep sense of the fact that there is an underlying meaning which the subject is always hoping or fearing to catch. The repeater of set phrases, on the other hand, looks for more illumination from what is familiar, or may have caught that spirit in language which regards words and phrases as in themselves endowed with magical qualities, magical being a word which expresses the dynamic aspect of symbolic efficacy.

The subject, let us suppose, merges the images of his waking thought-life in the words he more or less painfully learns to fit to them. Henceforward, economy favours the discontinuance of the habit of reviving mental images. But here again subjects must vary very considerably; with some the language habit will become a mere code, and with others it will remain a system which is alive with the original emotional picture elements. The latter will be " imaginative " subjects; the former, superficially more prosaic, will have the stream of ancient emotional experience flowing somewhere at a deeper level and expressing itself, or capable of expressing itself, in some other way, through actions involving grosser systems of musculature.

It is necessary to say something about the important emotional accompaniment of conceptual experience which is generally called " affect," but for which, as I said above, I prefer the term " symbolic efficacy." The word " affect " is too general. It is applicable to emotional manifestations at all stages, and emotion is thought of by students of psychology more particularly in immediate connection with the instincts. It is in connection with the instincts that emotion is first evolved in the life series. In the presence of the specific object of an instinct, whether one desired, as the worm by the robin for food, or one avoided, because an hereditary enemy, e.g., the hawk or owl by small birds generally, emotion of a positive or negative character promotes in the one case the search, in the other the escape. We see more clearly the effects of *negative* emotion ; fear, for instance, in human beings, is evinced by somatic disturbances, accelerated heart beat, sweating, pallor, etc. But *positive* emotion must be a fact no less, and probably bears a quantitative relation to the negative emotion expressed when the animal is thwarted in its pursuit. Who likes to take a bone from a hungry dog ? The anger which the thwarted dog shows must bear some sort of relation to the satisfaction which, for the dog, attends the meal. The positive emotion attending a discharge of energy wherever animal appetite is in question is an essential component of the emotional drive of the conceptual life which I call " Anxiety." The positive side of emotion, appetite, remains an enigma. It is literally occult. The other essential component of anxiety is negative emotion—fear or anger, or, in general, aversion. The positive and negative are so welded together in anxiety as to be often barely recognisable as one or the other. Conceptually speaking, these two originally attach, as I have endeavoured to show in Chapter II, to purely subjective situations; as the child in his conceptual life does not discriminate between the I and the Not-I, both negative and positive affects refer in the first instance to aspects of the self only. What is happening outside him is merely " stimulus." By Projection, anxiety is transferred later to objects outside the self, but always these objects are desired or feared in relation to the subjective life, even where emotion evoked on more primitive (perceptual) lines follows the same course. Thus, in positive attachments of an ordinary sexual character, the symbolic efficacy *and* the primitive sex drive of instinct both obviously act in unison. But that symbolic efficacy dominates the conceptual subject and is capable of deflecting emotion in him from the service of an instinct is seen in the case of obstinate sexual coldness. A subject of his own accord may dedicate himself to literal chastity. In the case of this subject, symbolic efficacy having made sexuality into an object to be feared, the ordinary attractiveness of the most desirable sex-object does not appear to exist for him ; the positive energy usually associated with the sex function is directed elsewhere and, as symbolic efficacy, advances some asexual object or pursuit into a means of salvation.

In concluding this chapter, a few words about Introjection in general may be in place. The best way, it would seem, to prevent abnormalities of instinct— for what applies to the sex appetite applies equally to the craving for food and to the normal desire for life itself, for amusement and excitement—is to teach our young people that no natural appetite is unclean or a thing of shame, but in itself something really beautiful, a manifestation of the Life-Principle.   Appetite is the " call of life."   When a child appears to be greedy or sexually inclined or excitable or ambitious, instead of scolding him and making him feel small, the better course would be to teach him to regard the life-urge in himself as something really wonderful and sacred which must not be expended wastefully or too exclusively (or indeed at all in the case of the sexual impulse) on immediate gratification, but reserved in part or wholly for uses much more elevated and more really satisfying than those to which the young subject, uninstructed, tends to put them.   To do this is to put the symbolic or sacramental aspect of life before him, and it is not to be thought that in doing this you are inculcating an attitude to life which is remote from your little child's own way of thinking.   Believe me, it is the primitive view the child himself takes of these matters.   It is the true one, to judge by the dream subject. *A too narrowly moral* attitude, equally with a *brutalising indifference* to the sacredness of the life-hunger, spoils the child's primitive sensitiveness. In the one case, he may, through sheer urge of instinct, arrive at a perverted interpretation of his own life-desire; in the other, through the insinuations of vicious persons his sensibility may become blunted to the exquisite beauty and delight which life when not divested of its symbolic values is capable of presenting for his enjoyment. Lack of opportunity to discuss these vital matters frankly and so to get to understand the " sacramental " is almost as serious for the developing conceptual subject as to discuss them with persons of a depraved turn of mind. If life is not sacramental for the conceptual subject, it is not capable of bringing him happiness worthy of the name.

Ordinary wisdom teaching to-day is miserably scrappy. There is an amusing illustration of this in the story of Rebecca of Sunnybrook Farm. The young heroine is desperately desirous of helping herself on the sly to some delicious dish, but in the act of lifting a spoonful to her mouth her eye falls on a motto containing a pious injunction relative to the enormity of dishonesty. She immediately relinquishes the desired morsel. As she is about to leave the scene of temptation, however, she catches sight of a further scrap of wisdom teaching, also framed and hanging on the wall for the enlightenment of the chance observer. This time she reads, " Heaven helps them who help themselves "; she returns triumphantly and secures the coveted mouthful. If our youth were trained on lines more really in accordance with the spirit of our historic teachers who spent themselves in the discussion of the inner meaning of the anxiety life and spared no pains to get at the full significance of the higher values of the life of the senses in which " as in a glass " we may see the reflection of the highest aspirations of the soul, there would be fewer broken hopes, fewer crimes against those we love best, fewer ruined lives.

There is too strong a tendency to-day to regulate introjection only with a view to the development of the practical moral subject, bread-winner, parent, citizen, etc. A utilitarian age tends to leave to chance all that is really of the greatest importance. In the *Psychology of Self-consciousness* I have attempted to show that, for happiness, life must be understood as a conceptual unity by the subject. Dogmatic teaching may do something, but mainly the subject must do the thing for himself under direction. I have attempted further to show that, in proportion to the want of unity in the subjective sphere, life will bring disillusionment, and not only so, but that want of unity is a positive source of physical, mental and moral danger.

More will not be said in this treatise about introjection, which is a side of the subject belonging to education and about which the dream psychologist can only frame conjectures. The rest of Part I of this treatise will be devoted to a discussion of Projection.

CHAPTER IV

PROJECTION

All the world's a stage and all the men and women merely players. (*As You Like It*)

LANGUAGE having reached a certain development, the vivid image-habit tends to fall into disuse in the waking life. Henceforward it is restricted, in so-called normal subjects, to the dream life, persons who are mediumistic or subject to hallucinations being regarded as abnormal.

Language expresses the conceptual subject's states of mind for all ordinary purposes. There are crises in life when language fails us, when we feel about language with John Donne, " Thou art too narrow and too weak to ease me now." On the whole, we prefer to feel like this as rarely as possible. Much stress is laid upon the importance of checking introspection ; how much stress is shown by the abhorrence with which people regard the habit of talking aloud when alone. We may think silently, although even this habit, regarded as desirable in special circumstances, is not looked upon with favour generally. Men that " think too much are dangerous," is Caesar's sentiment. Poets are regarded with a certain amount of suspicion so long as they are in the flesh. The impression is given that everything must be done to bring the subject out of himself, to make him live an active life in close touch with his fellows.

There is possibly a great conceptual truth involved here. " Saturated " anxiety, if I may use the term, *i.e.*, anxiety in which the two determinants are in a state of ideal equilibrium, may give little evidence externally of the marks which we associate with anxiety, and the idea may be that pressure will produce this desirable state. Projection of anxiety, as we shall see, serves so useful a purpose that there exists an over-determined tendency to insist on the projection of anxiety. All anxiety problems are required to express themselves in objective form. If we must have anxiety, the opinion prevails that it should take some intelligible shape ; one result of this is that colds, rheumatism, bilious attacks would seem to have more intelligibility than sorrow or repentance.

Disease, on the anxiety theory, is a bad habit the human race has acquired (together with many others) in its efforts to harmonise experience. Watching jealously over the attitude of the subject to existence on this globe, mankind by a consensus of opinion accepts disease as a legitimate projection of anxiety. The effect is to create a vicious circle. Disease has, to a certain extent, the effect of keeping the subject's attention riveted on material existence, but, since harmonisation of experience is the goal of the conceptual life, disease, like all anxiety manifestations, has also the effect of recalling the subjective attention to the inner aspect of life (" When the Devil was sick, the Devil a monk

would be."). In this *rôle*, disease is as much a
" flight from reality," *i.e.*, materialistic reality, as
the more definitely psycho-pathological manifestations of anxiety. But in sickness the " cheering
up " process, the inveterate habit we have of divert-
ing the invalid's attention from the problems which
have produced the sickness, again attempts to frus-
trate a beneficent provision of our constitution.

Projection is not made easy for the subject who
gives evidence of anxiety in other ways than disease,
especially if he has no material resources of his own.
He is then bandied from one callous charity system
to another. An anxiety subject in these circumstances complains bitterly of the difficulties of negotiating daily life. She compares the system to that
of Procrustes, the highwayman of Attica, who made
his involuntary visitors fit the one bed he had provided, instead of providing beds which fitted them.
If they were too long, he chopped off a part of them;
if too short, he put them on the rack to make them
longer.

The result of disregarding the anxiety problem is
that the subjective life tends to shrink back into the
dream whence it issued. When we go to bed, the
emotional problems which we cannot project, as
they are not allowed standing-room in consciousness, meet us again in dreams. Dreams, perhaps,
seem very unimportant in the life of most people.
I understand that this is not always the case. Dream
books exist and some simple people make a practice
of referring to such little dictionaries of symbolism.
I am not acquainted with books of the kind, possibly

they teach more truth than I am aware. A friend tells me that she has met among uneducated people those over whom the dream manual exercises a kind of tyranny. She has heard a woman, for instance, say that she has " them horrible feelings again," having dreamed of fish, and that had she in the dream identified herself with the fish, she would not have ventured out of the house! Someone is informed that there has been a row. " Oh! don't tell me that," is the rejoinder, "I dreamt of photos" (and therefore expected a row).

Until recently, when it has become the fashion to discuss dreams, to give attention to dreams would have seemed extremely superstitious and that would have been enough to damn it, as everybody is afraid of being superstitious. But a Roman gentleman was not. Horace tells us that if you meet an object regarded as ill-omened, when leaving the house, you must not venture out the same morning. The word superstition (*super-sto*) means " standing over." What can this word mean if not that a mood comes on us which makes us pause and pay some respect, long overdue, to the anxiety life within? Something in the experience of sense has struck a chord which reverberates in the subjective life; our attention is arrested and we halt and " stand over " the problem. The outward and visible sign may be a mere prescription common to the group of which the subject is a member, e.g., to turn the money in your pocket on seeing the new moon; or it may be an idiosyncrasy of the subject; most people have their special superstitions and most people laugh

over them. A moment when superstition seriously
assails us is one, generally, when we are in straits of
any sort. Nervous symptoms are related to superstition.

We cannot get away from the anxiety life, it rules
us, and it rules us through our experience of the
night, whether we dream or not, perhaps even
whether we sleep or not. The dream revives the
ancient infantile habit of feeling and thinking in
images, and the images are replenished from
present-day experience which has symbolic efficacy
of any degree. Dream images are symbols, and, in
these days, to have full practical use, dreams must
be interpreted; through them we may then learn
what in the inner life is our attitude to things really.
In any case, the dream, quite unknown to us, tends
to govern our waking hours—we project it. The
regulative function of the dream for waking life is
not suspected by most people and is not made any
point of by most dream psychologists.

None the less the dreams of adulthood still function as the primitive mental images of childhood
did. They are dynamic on account of symbolic
efficacy and create dramatic situations, or, in other
words (as Professor Freud), they prefigure experience in waking life not only remotely, but in detail
and all the time. The dream is not the end-effect;
quite the contrary. The dreamer awakens with delayed motor reactions seeking an outlet which will
cause the subject to create situations in his waking
life, as the child creates them in his play. Since
the dream comes to consciousness in symbols, and

we do not trouble to interpret it, it is the symbolism and not the latent reality which tends to reach expression and rule the reactions of waking life. Here is the crux of the conceptual life. A condition of sanity is that the projections of the dream state adapt themselves to the limits imposed by morality and rationality. This condition is often very difficult to fulfil. Sometimes it is done only by damping down anxiety. The anxiety subject who feels himself in danger of projecting symbols which are taboo in his group will restrict Introjection and Projection, being satisfied to live only in humdrum situations; or he takes drugs or drink or indulges in long hours of sleep. The anxiety subject in a crisis must be kept quiet on this same account and, if necessary, controlled by sedatives, in case he create Projection situations which will furnish fresh material for Introjection.

In all cases, as the dreamer has no knowledge of the symbolic nature of his dreams, he is tempted to take the dream symbolism literally. The fact that he probably forgets his dream on waking prevents his recognising the source of the particular urge he is aware of in the morning. " I have been thinking," more often than not means " I have been dreaming," and it is in the morning that the new thoughts present themselves. Not to understand the dream as a symbol lands us in the same place as we should find ourselves in, if we interpreted literally the symbolism embodied in the language of every day. I am reminded of a foolish little Christy Minstrel joke which illustrates this. " I was given a sum of money by my kind old father, who says ' put it away for a rainy day, my boy.' It rained the next day and I spent the lot," concludes the punster.

To project the symbol literally leads to three aspects of projection :

1. There is the *practical* aspect of projection. We are so accustomed to think of mind function as the function of the waking mind that we wonder sometimes at the subtlety and intelligence displayed by the mind in sleep. This is only revealed fully on analysis, for the manifest content of the dream is often a poor motley affair, a mere patchwork, and it is only through investigation that the beautiful dream work is discovered. Nevertheless, even so the dream picture often brings together material in such a way as to be suggestive. One can believe that practical suggestions have often been conveyed by dreams with full knowledge of the dreamer. The dreamer sees himself, his clothing or his abode, or some part of them, with certain additions or differences of arrangement, and his attention is brought back to practical matters which may have escaped him. Again, he meets in the dream acquaintances he has not seen for a long time and interests and occupations of former times are recalled. Hence kindly thought or disfavour is directed to persons long forgotten. The results of this process may be good or bad, but they act alike in focussing attention on persons and concerns which are matters of ordinary interests; one can well believe that, through dreams, human institutions

have come into being, and, having come, have established themselves in common use.

2. The dreamer may chance to have presented to him in the dream unusual and beautiful material —a beautiful landscape, a lovely person or an unusually attractive object. This experience will probably have an elevating effect on him. In this case his projection has what is called an *anagogic,* or upwards-leading, effect. The tone of his whole mind is raised by contemplation of the aesthetic composition. Sometimes, because the material introjected is sordid or unpleasant, by *reaction* the dreamer is rendered more scrupulous.

3. On the other hand, the dream may exercise a *catagogic* or downwards-leading tendency. Dreams having a manifest content of the kind last mentioned often synchronise with an indifference to the minor decencies. Habits in relation to expenditure, to punctuality and order, as well as some forms of perverted self-expression, being lineally descended from infantile preoccupation with the bodily functions, are introduced into the dream with the greatest freedom of treatment. The real significance of these symbols is unknown to the dreamer, and because attention is directed towards them in the form in which they present themselves, they acquire undue prominence and keep the subject a slave to the trivial and incidental, or possibly worse. Speaking quite generally, if the higher life which makes itself felt through the dream, by means often of strangely unlovely analogies, does not receive its due, it will, by the very irritation which confusion

D

engenders, keep the attention of the subject riveted on objects and interests which are far from elevating. The highest interests must be served, or ritual, in the shape of perverted habits, will be invented, and the chances are that, without conscious control, the tendency will be downwards and not upwards. Conscious control dictates that the higher life-interests be remembered and served by a carefully chosen ritual of sacramental efficacy; acknowledgment of the All-of-Life in prayer and thanksgiving and of dependence thereon in grace before meat and intercession at special seasons; commemoration of the festivals of dear discarnate spirits, as well as of those living in our midst; recognition of the sacredness of family ties and of all sacred relations—these it is which satisfy the inner life of man and provide the sacred chain on which the pearls of contentment and sustained effort are threaded. Failing them, the young subject will invent ways of serving his deity, *i.e.,* of expressing anxiety, and in the case of the majority, these inventions, through the sheer urgency of the familiar symbol, will exhibit a tendency to revert to the baseness of savagery or the triviality of infancy.

The two following chapters will deal with the most common classes of dream symbolism and an attempt will be made to show how, while the inner teaching of the humblest dream symbol is exquisitely lofty, through its direct and literal projection the light which is in Man may become darkness.

CHAPTER V

THE MESSAGE OF SYMBOLISM

A primrose by the river's brim
A yellow primrose was to him,
And it was nothing more.
(Peter Bell, Wordsworth)

To me the meanest flower that blows can give
Thoughts that do often lie too deep for tears.
(Intimations of Immortality, Wordsworth)

IT is true that so many of us are indifferent to what
this wonderful world, which we call the natural
world, is.   If we feel the need to understand what is
involved even in a single primrose we are fairly on
our way in the search for the purpose of life.   This
little structure, the primrose, has been built up by
the Life-Principle through the bringing together
of various inorganic elements and the mixing in
therewith of the Life-Principle itself to provide
what are called organic substances.   These, by laws
as immutable as those which govern the succession of day and night, produce the beautiful harmony of plant, leaf and flower which we know as
the primrose. According to the estimates of science,
it took the Life-Principle an incredibly long time, as
we count time, to gather together in its laboratory
the material and the tools requisite for producing
the primrose.   In the geological series, in which, as
in a book, all the members of man and everything

appertaining thereto are written, the order to which the primrose belongs appears late among fossil remains of plants. When human parents expect their baby, they make great preparations; the nursery, the cradle, the tiny garments, etc., are all thought out long before their little owner comes to claim them. So the Life-Principle created on this globe conditions which made it a world exquisitely suited for its most highly-favoured sons and daughters—men and women. The process of preparation is called Interadaptation.

Dr. Caldecott says (*The Philosophy of Religion*, p. 22) :—

> There are instances of things which seem to have a purpose to fulfil over and above their intrinsic being; effects to produce on other things from which, in some cases, a reciprocal action proceeds to themselves, e.g., the relation of the plant kingdom to the animal; there is at least an appearance of this correlation having been in the view of whatever may be supposed to be the power or powers which have operated to produce them.

The vegetable world paves the way for the animal kingdom, because the plant can subsist on *inorganic* particles, whereas for animal subsistence *organic* particles are necessary. In animals, the Life-Principle became flesh and one after another the different species appeared, each in turn exhibiting new possibilities, both in regard to organic function and psychological manifestation. The incredible beauty of this process seems to some marred by the fact that it is necessary for the higher species to live through the perishing of the lower. Animal life feeds on plant life and one animal species makes prey of another species. Man himself is in some respects the most cruel of all. As Man comes to know the laws of his own life it will come about that he will learn also to introduce into this world justice and harmony, not only for the enjoyment of his own kind, but for that of all living things besides. The old anthropocentric doctrine, the doctrine which represents the earth as the centre of the universe and man himself as the centre of every interest on the earth, is, supposedly, long ago exploded, but in a sense there is truth in it, at any rate so far as the second part of the doctrine is concerned. Man is obviously the climax of the efforts of the Life-Principle on this globe and he is responsible for all here. He has been given dominion over the fish of the sea and the fowls of the air.

Dominion is his in virtue of the fact that he re-presents a new departure. He is a new creature whom self-consciousness has quickened. The human foetus, a teeming mass of primitive cells, gradually assumes in the mother's womb forms which distantly recall, stage by stage, the develop-ment of animal life on this globe. At a certain time this mass is " quickened," made alive as a whole unified being, and the animal man is there; the baby moves and kicks and starts on his new life. Born into the world a little perceptual subject, he lies there curiously unlike the offspring of every other species, singularly helpless, that the condi-tions may be fulfilled for a further development of

life. Helplessness, the cutting off of energy from
all motor channels, is necessary for a considerable
period that energy may accumulate and make a condition such that the specifically human element shall
come to be. Man is " quickened " anew into self-
consciousness. Henceforward he lives not to himself but to the Life or God principle within, and,
for the attainment of his spiritual majority, he must
knock up against all the objects in his great nursery,
the world, that he may learn to project what of God
is in his inner consciousness and recreate the world
in thought.

I have suggested above that Anxiety in the unconscious provides a mechanism for this evolution
of mind. In anxiety, as in a mirror, the experience
of terrestrial conditions is *reflected*. The incoming
process I have called Introjection and the outgoing
process Projection. Introjected material finds a
place in the unconscious because it provides a picture or symbol, derived from without, of anxiety
processes within; at the same time energy is trans-
muted, *i.e.,* *de*tached from the material and
*at*tached to the symbol. The symbol retains its
grasp on waking consciousness on account of its
symbolic efficacy and, on its pattern, humanity
maps out the material world and creates an ordered
universe which reflects the purposes and ordinances
of the All-of-Life. The conceptual apparatus, of
which the dream is part, is the Imagination, and in
it, as in a mirror, the things of sense are reflected.
It is a magic mirror, a mirror which adds something
to the picture.

We must now look at the symbols themselves and see if we can read something of their immediate meaning. I have said elsewhere (Chap. II, pp. 12 *et seq.*) that the symbols first created are those which convey emotional states. They originate in mental pictures which may in the first instance be faces. The child is suddenly countered by an angry parent whose face and gestures convey the impression of displeasure; again, the pleased face and winning gestures stand out in contrast to the above. In the new sphere of experience thus created, the child cannot at first discriminate between that which is within and that which is without, so the visual image is in the first instance referred within, for it is obviously a subjective experience.

These early picture faces must convey what is extremely painful or pleasurable. I remember personally as a child of about eight or nine, when suffering from a slight attack of fever, that I had a recurrence of such images in a night dream. They caused great terror. The faces came nearer and then receded. I can only describe them as *faces,* for there was nothing about them by which they could be associated with any person. When revived in memory at the present day, they bring with them detailed impressions of the exact place where the dream occurred. The dream and experiences associated with it survive even at this distance of time on account of the symbolic efficacy. Dreams commonly are full of the images of persons. We are safe in assuming that persons in the dream stand for emotional states and mental attitudes. If we could doubt this from the evidence of the dream, which is overwhelmingly in favour of such an interpretation, we have the evidence of language. Person (*persona*) means mask. In classical drama actors wore masks, every role being well defined. The old man or the head of the family, the young man or lover, and the slave, each was known to the audience by the mask which the actor taking the part put on. It was assumed that certain mental characteristics went along with each mask. Probably every dreamer has, on the same principle, an original set of *dramatis personae* among the stage properties of his own dream life, but the originals are rarely brought to light; they are relegated to some dark corner as being too painfully primitive, and their places are taken by a succession of surrogates or representatives. Through the Introjection process, the bald simplicity of the terrifying face is subdued and furnished with many subsidiary details of dress and posture. These latter at once modify and particularise further the emotional content of the original types; mother, father, brothers, sisters, and a few additional stereotyped characters hold their own, as a rule, in most people's dreams amid an otherwise shifting dream population. Dreamers vary extraordinarily in the number of persons they are capable of introjecting. As everything in the dream is the dreamer, the greater the number of dream population the higher has been the degree of the passive analysis of experience of the particular subject in early life, we may suppose. A dream given to me once represented the poor dream subject surrounded by all the population of Madame Tussaud's famous exhibition, all pressing round him with evidences of curiosity and interest but in utter silence.   The dreamer described it as an awful nightmare.   I think the number and variety of the persons represented reflected the dreamer's strongly developed introspective tendency in childhood, and their silence, the absence of power to express or to organise his anxiety life.   Such a subject seems to have lacked as a child the gift of protecting his conceptual life from intrusion.   His sensitive mind, as a little child, had an absorbent quality which rendered him the prey of every passing impression, whereas a child more favourably circumstanced would through the activities of play introduce greater organisation into his conceptual life and exclude therefrom all elements not having a certain degree of intelligibility for him.

Persons in the dream represent mental characteristics on the same principle that the old morality plays introduced Envy, Greed, Curiosity, etc., etc., as separate personalities.   Parts of the body no less may represent abstract ideas or conceptual values. Vital organs figure more particularly.   The heart, for instance, may stand for the central driving power, the conceptual possibilities of the subject as a whole ; the head for his power of control, for his thinking possibilities or his self-respect ; the hand for his active principle, etc. ; eyes and ears receive messages transmitted to him from other souls. Literature makes use freely of such figures—the

heart bowed down with woe, the heart desperately
wicked; the head held up, covered, etc.; the hand
cut off, restricted by bonds, raised in abjuration;
eyes and ears that can or cannot see or hear.

We have supposed that the little child only gradually comes to a knowledge of a mind-self, unseen,
operating through the body as its instrument.   No
one troubles to teach him about this.   He is called
good or naughty and he naturally supposes that it
is the offending member of his body with which the
sin originates.   In the psychological literature I
think of a quaint story told of a small boy who com-
plained that his fingers, contrary to instruction,
would not desist from picking his nose.   He, the
subject, disclaimed with naivete all responsibility
for the action of his hand.   Nevertheless, the
unseen mind-self is well known to the dream, but,
the dream symbol being the body, the dreamer's
waking consciousness does not probe further and
the child's crude materialism is never corrected.
The dream depicts a person, and a concreteness,
entirely foreign to the dream's meaning, attaches
itself forthwith to that dream element.   Johnny may
stand for a lying tendency or Tommy for a taste for
ill-gotten gains, but the dreamer has no notion of
this in the morning.   He laughs over his dreams as
a rule, not because they are necessarily humorous,
but, he will tell you, because they are so " funny,"
so unexpected, often quaint, with a certain incongruity which excites his sense of the ridiculous.

The great principle of symbolism is that human
bodies, their parts and functions, as the equivalent

of the mind and its attributes, constitute the first class of symbols. In the dream everything, of course, refers to the dreamer, but the history of the introjection of every dream element is, as a rule, easily provided by association.

Around the above principle, as the central nucleus of symbolism, other classes of symbols arise. The habit of the dream remains very largely symbolic and with new experience the new material introjected may be applied to bring out more and more precisely the spiritual lesson. The inference suggests itself that range and vividness of perceptual experience, other things being equal, enrich the self-consciousness within. It has always been remarked that in mental disorders the latest inventions of the human race are laid under contribution in the attempt to give more adequate utterance to something which in the subject is endeavouring to reach expression. Bizarre as a jargon of atoms, electrons, flying machines, poisonous gases and wireless telephony may seem to the observer, there is an important principle involved. An analogy is always more dynamic while it is fresh. As the freshness wears off, unless it is a particularly elevated symbol, capable of being appreciated by the reflecting person, or, failing this, expressed in language of great beauty, we say it is hackneyed or trite. Great stress in these matters is laid on originality, as that shows that the suggestion springs directly from the subject's living psychic sources and is not a mere imitation.

For dream purposes the mind must be furnished,

provided with a location and seen in relation to experience generally. Clothing and buildings and other appliances of man's invention, as symbols, express these things from different aspects. Clothing hides the body and at the same time expresses it; in the dream it represents in general the subject's reactions to vital situations. This is natural, for our clothing varies according to the occasion, sometimes we wear a workaday dress and again on special occasions we wear something more elaborate. The dream abounds in such symbolism. In the parable of the wedding guest without a wedding garment the idea is conveyed exactly; the word " turncoat " gives another aspect of the symbol. Functionaries of every kind are known by their particular costume; the policeman, for instance, and the soldier are both familiar dream figures.

Among all articles of attire the hat perhaps occurs most insistently and is always deserving of attention. It appears to symbolise the way of thinking,[1] the controlling attitude to experience, perhaps. A change of hat marks a change in one's way of thinking; to be hatless is perhaps to be fancy free. Through the dream one catches a glimpse of the educational value of clothing. The emphasis laid on the toilet can easily be overdone, but, equally, indifference to the toilet can be harmful.

---

[1] The following has been brought to my notice :—
" I will not keep this form upon my head (*tearing off her head-dress*)
While there is such disorder in my wit."
(*King John III*, 4)

Another class of symbolism provides the unseen self with a habitation. The mind is attached to the body; symbols required to express this relation are supplied by buildings of various kinds; by objects, that is to say, which bear the same relation to the body (the symbol of the mind) which the body does to the mind. " I am in a house," or " indoors," is a common dream feature; indeed, as is implied by the dreamer's direct statement of the fact, there is an important difference involved in the fact of dreaming you are in a house and dreaming you are in the open. General literature is full of the same imagery, which is obviously natural when the main nuclear symbol, Body =Soul, is once understood : the body is the " temple of the living God " (the Life-Principle); the " soul's dark cottage." Examples could easily be multiplied; in allegorical literature we have many passages where this figure is carried out in detail, *e.g.,* Spenser's *Faery Queene,* Book II, Canto 10.

Useful articles of man's invention as the equivalent for parts of the body is perhaps a little more difficult to realise; nevertheless, the fact is established by the study both of the dream and of general literature. In the dream, for instance, pots and kettles occur as organs or even tissues in which metabolic changes take place; these—both utensils and tissues—wear out sometimes and waste accumulates, awaiting elimination. Metabolic processes, as processes of combustion, are suitably symbolised by burning. The body is a kitchen or chemical laboratory. When the process is healthful, the fire is under control; when pathological, the fire is a destructive one, but the fabric is not necessarily suffering damage, there may be only a consumption of waste going on. Another and higher expression of energy manifestation is light.

Chair, bed, etc., symbolise the parts of the body which come into contact with these pieces of furniture; the table is the female reproductive organ; soft furnishings, pillows, eiderdowns, cloths of all kinds are the soft tissues. Sometimes these are represented as having rents and patches, or other defects. The knowledge which the dream mind possesses of somatic states is almost incredible. Probably years before the onset of a disease, the picture thereof may be deposited in the gallery of dream symbols of the particular subject.[1]

One important class of dream symbols relates to the second mental subject which resides in the economy of every one of us, the perceptual or animal subject. This is appropriately expressed by animals. The perceptual subject is, as a general rule, dominated by the higher subject and the reactions to this domination of the junior partner are conveyed to the consciousness of the higher through the dream. The biting animal is often the perceptual subject in revolt. Elaborate dreams in which the dream subject is represented as attacked by cat or by dog, which bites him often in the hand, the active principle, are common and are generally attended by great fear. Another recalcitrant animal is the ass. Sometimes the animal is in distress or

[1] But the disease-picture must never be interpreted literally.

in difficulties. The animal chosen, together with his condition and his attitude to the dream subject, are each and all of importance down to the veriest detail. The half-human, half-animal dream element suggests energy only in part redeemed for the service of the conceptual life. Again, literature and folk-lore abound with such; some innocent and pathetic, like mermaid and merman; others more or less hideous, like minotaur, centaur and satyr. The subject in whom such monsters occur has not, by high thinking and low living, brought his energy up to the higher nervous centres, or, in the language of the dream, he dwells in a lower storey of the house. The staircase with its various levels seems to represent this difference in location of energy.

There are various other classes of dream symbolism and some objects enter into two or more classes. When we find out the dream meaning we always discover unerring analogical accuracy. Travelling is a common symbol; every variety of locomotion, passive or active, has its exact interpretation in every individual case and always has ultimately to do with the main theme of the dream—Salvation. But the immediate application may be entirely concrete and refer to the body, *e.g.,* to the circulation or to the peristalsis.

The vegetable world supplies symbolism which has an equal if not a superior width of range. Our most cherished flower, the rose, for instance, may mean anything connected with the great determinant expiation, from self-giving in the abstract to

bleeding in particular. Growing things may symbolise growth in holiness or growths in the tissues.
The spiritual interpretation is the desideratum, but
our habits of thought call our attention more
particularly to the physical. The body is a link in
the chain, a link supremely important for every
reason.

In fine, a discussion of dream symbolism to be
exhaustive would be a complete compendium of
human interests and concerns, from the highest to
the lowest. Only sheer limitation of space would
bring any treatise on the subject to a close. Symbolism is at once rigidly fixed in principle and
infinitely varied and flexible in application and in
detail. The dream, the apparatus which reflects
the deep purposes of the Life-Principle within,
whose manifestations we too often twist and distort
in a thousand ways, is capable, I believe, of acting
as the subject's faithful cicerone and guide. From
point to point in experience, every introjected element could be built into the fabric of immortality;
and again, through intelligent projection it would
become the means of illuminating the next step.
Happy would such an one be to use terrestrial
experience; he would not divorce contemplation and
action, but with courage and sagacity husband his
spiritual resources in the darkness and stillness of
the season of growth, and again be able and willing
to pay out, if need were, in lavish self-sacrifice. The
practice of sacramental living is an art which has
yet to be acquired by the majority of mankind.

CHAPTER VI

HOW THE SYMBOL CAN MAKE OR MAR LIFE

Look not thou down but up !
To uses of a cup,
The festal board, lamp's flash and trumpet's peal,
The new wine's foaming flow,
The master's lips a-glow !
Thou, heaven's consummate cup, what need'st thou with earth's
wheel ?

(Rabbi ben Ezra, R. Browning)

HUMAN life, as we have seen in Chapter IV, is speaking generally, a projection of the dream on waking experience. This is true both of the race (phylogenetically, as it is called), and of the individual (or ontogenetically). The real meaning of the symbol reaches us sometimes through the channel of religion and the arts, but, for the most part, unless our lives allow a place for these more elevated concerns, the symbol introjected is bald and paltry and it carries our interests little beyond itself. Being a symbol, it carries symbolic efficacy and hence assures attention for itself, provided always that the symbolic efficacy is of a degree that can be tolerated. Symbols to which a high degree of symbolic efficacy attaches may seem " dirty " or unpleasant or terrible, and will tend to be dismissed with a laugh or a shudder.

There is a personal coefficient to be taken into account here, for the symbolic efficacy attaching to

E

any particular symbol is sometimes greater for one individual than for others. Eating is an example of this. Nervous people cannot always eat before others and in some disordered mental states the subject even has the idea that he should not eat at all. Others, again, are greedy. Symbolic efficacy for all these people attaches to eating in a higher degree than it does to most people. The merely nervous person may not be able to account for his idiosyncrasy at all; the "unbalanced" subject, on the other hand, who refuses to eat, will allege reasons which will convince no one; people will probably, in the name of charity, subject him to the torture of forcible feeding.

The direct projection of the symbol has had many useful consequences, as is obvious when it is realised that human culture has been built up thereby. The symbolism of the original primitive equation, Body = Soul, has, for instance, rendered mankind valuable practical service. It ensures that we shall take care of our bodies; keep them clean and beautiful and healthy; clothe and feed them suitably; and generally cherish them. The same thing applies to the house which in the dream stands for the body. As we care for the body because it is a symbol of the soul, so we care for our habitation because it is the symbol of the body. Some people are more concerned for their houses than for their persons; their furniture must be carefully planned, every article in keeping; or it must be kept in a perfect condition, for this reflects the harmony which they wish to see in the organs of the body. Again, we choose our pastimes and games, urged thereto by introjected remnants of experience, which survive to provide dream symbolism out of all the many and varied pursuits and interests which encounter us in daily life. Ball games enjoy a special prestige, because this object, by its spherical shape, easily lends itself as a symbol for the immortal self bandied about between the opposite determinants of anxiety (see Part II, the Anxiety Drama), or perhaps between the claims of the two opposite modes of experience, perceptual and conceptual.

The direct and literal projection of dream symbolism works, in fact, in the direction of regulating human life, and when it does this it is most valuable, providing that it does not exclude the higher interests which lie behind the symbolism. This is no mean danger. The practical attitude to the concerns of human life having been fostered for generations of human culture, the memory of their symbolic origin has been to a great extent lost; indeed, the " hard-headed " person prides himself on taking them just as they present themselves to him, as ordinary matters, the interest of which begins and ends with themselves. He loses the sacramental view of life and will think and act on utilitarian principles alone. The danger which threatens this man is that he may bring into the same category everything which pertains to life, the more remote and sacred as well as the commonplace and trivial. He will argue that his needs and impulses are " natural " and may be indulged so long as the laws of hygiene are obeyed, also that his relations with other men are, in general, similar to those of the lower animals, but regulated by rules of social expediency which reason dictates. It was such a temper of mind that evolved *Emile* and the *Contrat Social*. The claims of anxiety are set aside ; in the waking life man makes himself a petty king in a materialistic universe. He becomes the devotee of Reason. Reason is a good prime minister to the Life Principle, but under the regime of Reason as usurper of the supreme power there lurk serious dangers. [1]

The dangerous aspect of projecting the symbol literally becomes easily apparent when, one symbol-system having been singled out, the symbolic efficacy gathers momentum and concentrates upon this particular outlet for anxiety. Whatever we call it, we then have a psycho-neurosis to deal with. For instance, anxiety may be precipitated on the *body,* the symbol of the soul, in the form of disease. The disease is at once a picture of the supposed state of the soul and the means of the punishment thereof. The majority of our most detestable complaints probably originates thus. Cancer, adolescent decline, heart disease, etc., etc., are not generally thought to have such an origin, but the study of anxiety provides ample evidence that they have. The *essential causes* of specifically human diseases must be sought outside the physiological series. The bodies of men and women are, it is true, the most wonderful " adaptive mechanisms "

[1] See Appendix I. No. 2.

which the Life-Principle has built up,[1] but Anxiety frustrates the very optimism of nature and turns her tools into lethal weapons.   Anxiety, like any other jealous governor, may resuscitate out-of-date statutes to reinforce its decrees.   We must never forget that for the dream subject the body is only environment.

Similarly, anxiety may develop an attitude of uneasiness towards every trifling defect in the *house,* the symbol of the body.   A certain subject, for instance, cannot resist worrying over and attempting to remove every little speck which she detects on her walls or furniture.   Her mind is obsessed all the time by such spots and defects and she is much distressed.   The dreams of this subject show that in the symbolism the emphasis has been laid at a formative period on the equation House = Body, probably to relieve anxiety.   It has not had, as a matter of fact, the desired effect, but her trouble is transferred to the mental sphere.   The dangers of literal projection suggest the need for the cultivation of a different attitude to the problems of the inner life.   The symbolic aspect of human life must be understood, especially this deep and firmly-rooted equation, Body = Soul and all that flows therefrom.

Education, having recognised the fact that *energy follows attention,* will come to occupy itself more seriously with the question of *balance of interest.*   Before all things, there must be a balance established   between   conceptual   and   perceptual

[1] Crile, *Man an Adaptive Mechanism.*

interests. It is essential for health and happiness.
The sacramental character of material existence
must never be lost sight of, for this is what is
characteristically human in our mental make-up; it
is the essence of culture. Man must always fail
under the strain involved in neglecting one or other
side of his dual nature. The individual is sure to
break down sooner or later in body or mind, or to
become depraved in character unless he is taught
more consistently the structure and meaning of his
own thought-life. Balance is characteristic of
healthy life. In former days sanity and health were
safe-guarded by the fact that men and women lived
far less strenuously than at present and that they
considered it good form to observe the Sunday and
certain religious exercises. It is true that many
forgot from Monday to Saturday what occupied
them on Sunday, a defect which brings its own
aftermath of suffering and which requires its particular remedy.

Examples have been given illustrating Anxiety
as disease-bearer in the bodily and mental spheres
respectively. There are other direct or literal projections of the symbolism which results in depravity
of character. The association in the symbolism of
Sexuality and Death, derived from the major equation Body$=$Soul, may be regarded as the source
of sexual mania and also of sadism and masochism.
Aggressive sexuality and violence appear from the
dream to be convertible terms. The process in the
unconscious which produced the symptom known
as sadism may be something like the following:

the conceptual subject is overweighted with a sense of the need for expiation. He *will not,* or perhaps he *cannot* bear it himself; he must therefore find a substitute or substitutes. Thus referred, expiation finds a vent as aggressive sexuality or cruelty. In a case when an obsessive sense of sin is not referred, the subject seeks suffering, self-inflicted or inflicted by another.

It is unnecessary to labour technical details further. Psychological re-education illuminates for the individual the unconscious bye-ways where this symbolism has its stronghold, and not only prevents its direct application, but presents the full picture of the symbolism together with its true interpretation. Conviction comes, as a rule, only with the evolution of the dreamer's own Anxiety drama, but sane teaching on the true facts of the conceptual life goes far to prepare the way.

Is the judgment which mankind has passed on the psycho-neurotic just? Is he a slacker? Does he hug his sin and allow fear, detached from this, the original source, to attach itself to indifferent objects? If this is a well-founded charge, and it may be so in many cases, the subject is not, at any rate as a rule, a conscious defaulter. During the period when the apparatus of self-consciousness is developing within him, during the first years of life, that is to say, he is quite helpless in regard to the introjection process. It is then that the most obstinate mental habits of the conceptual life are formed. The main onus of the responsibility cannot therefore fairly rest with the subject, but must be accepted by the child's guardians and educators.

To take one or two examples illustrating the danger which attends the direct application of dream symbolism.   These examples will at the same time illustrate the clarifying effect on the mind of the true interpretation.   A youth brings a dream in which he sees a parade of soldiers; large numbers of them march by in orderly fashion; at the end the Field-Marshal approaches the dreamer and shakes hands with him.   The psychology of the young dreamer is well known to me.   His mind has been full of conflict, some of which is lightened, with the result that he is developing satisfactorily in mind and physique.   Uninstructed even at this stage, he regards his dream in the ordinary negligent fashion and takes soldiers and Field-Marshal at their familiar values.   His interest in soldiers is thereby heightened for the moment and he even talks of enlisting, a course of action which would be decidedly premature.   A little touch of gratified vanity sounds in his voice as he relates the incident of the Commanding Officer's courtesy towards himself.   I brush such flimsy interpretations on one side.   I ask him what soldiers and Commander, respectively, stand for in symbolism.   I then congratulate him on the dream picture, which presents to him his vital fighting forces in perfect order and discipline, obedient to their superior officers, the chief of whom is in accord with the young dream subject.   The dream so interpreted is a true description of the young man, in spite of the serious nervous breakdown which brought him under our care a comparatively short time ago.   He was then so broken down physically and mentally that I felt a pardonable anxiety at the sight of him.   He now presents the picture of a well-set-up and frank-faced youth.   About the same time the same subject brought another dream, the manifest content of which was as unlike the above as it is well possible for the two dreams to be.   He showed considerable embarrassment at first, said it was a " rotten dream " and postponed the moment of recital.   I reminded him that dream pictures were symbols and that their meaning was always quite different from the manifest content.   So exhorted, he told his dream.   The very simple dream picture, it turned out, was that his mother was about to have a baby ! I reminded him of the previous dream of the soldiers and pointed out to him that this one, although in its outward seeming so strangely different, was, as a matter of fact, capable of being linked up with it in meaning.   The mother is the symbol of self-giving, and the baby, the future promise of life, the symbol of the soul.   The selfish boy develops into the man, who, as opportunity offers, will take on the responsibilities of life in a generous spirit and become a soul subject, finally winning the laurels of immortality.   The effect on this youth of his own dream, in spite of its really elevating meaning, would, on the lines of any other dream theory, have had a debasing effect, feeding a puerile curiosity and re-enforcing a morbid attitude to sex.   Like all biological material, and

that in the highest degree, since it is the heart of
the mystery of the conceptual life, sex considera-
tions must be taken at one and the same time in the
spirit of simple common sense and also in the spirit
of deepest reverence. With the right understanding of his dreams the youthful subject leaves the
psychologist's room with smiling eyes and hope in
his heart. What seemed to him base has become
ennobled. He realises that the conceptual life is a
human life and he is advanced in his possession of
what is the greatest heritage of humanity, our great
common thought life. By slow degrees he will
learn that the conceptual subject is bi-sexual and
why this is so, and he will not be tempted, as he
undoubtedly otherwise might be tempted by such
dreams, to turn aside into the paths of sexual per-
version, but will instead soften, with gracious
human charity, a mind of excellent possibilities and
genuinely masculine.

" Look not thou down but up ! "

The "catagogic" tendency must be withstood ; the
conceptual life is worse and more unhappy in every
way than the sheer animal's if it be not an upward-
looking life. The conceptual subject's conversation is in Heaven, and Heaven is in the first place
within and in the second place in a community of
other conceptual subjects. " *Thou, Heaven's
consummate cup, what need'st thou with earth's
wheel?* " The cup, the conceptual subject, says
Browning in effect, is for eternity; " potter and

clay endure." " The Wheel," *i.e.*, the conditions
of time, space and matter, is

>Machinery, just meant
>To give thy soul its bent,
>Try thee and turn thee forth sufficiently impressed.

A word is in place here about the ordinary
methods of dream interpretation. Through an
inconsistent application of the law of symbolism of
dreams propounded by Professor Freud, the common practice of dream psychologists leads to a re-
enforcement of the dangerous habit of taking the
manifest content of the dream literally. The " bio-
logic " interpretation of the dream is a positive
menace to society, for in the name of authority and
science it sanctions concentration on the manifest
content in an even higher degree than would
happen if the subject were uninstructed. Energy
follows attention and the result is a rapid decentralisation of symbolic efficacy. This reverses the plan
of man's evolution; the subject is encouraged to
rush into a vain attempt to satisfy along sensuous
channels the urge of life which is really calling him
along the higher path. If the method succeeds, it
is a doubtful cure to exchange the higher for the
lower. The more sensitive psyche will either collapse in despair in the process or anxiety will work
a speedy revenge on the subject in terms of physical
disability.

CHAPTER VII

THE PROJECTION OF EMOTION

Set a thief to catch a thief.

(*Proverb*)

I have said that the dream is like a mirror upon which fall the images of passing events to be reflected (or projected) on to experience again. But the mirror is a magic mirror. It is a *transmuter of energy;* a delicate piece of mechanism capable of converting the concrete happening introjected into a vehicle for expressing the deeper and more mysterious values of consciousness or feeling. It is here, as I have said, that we touch the occult. [1] Bodily states we can describe, but not consciousness, not feeling, not pain, not pleasure, still less anxiety, remorse or ecstasy. In vain the psychologist describes *behaviour;* this is only the outside shell, the mechanism; the substance, the reality behind, remains a mystery. It is a mystery of the Life-Principle — the Unknowable in Spencer's phrase. [2]

That which is describable, the symbol of the mystery, the material reality, is vehicle only. Emotional consciousness, the higher reality, is indescribable.

[1] " Hearing, seeing, touch and the power to communicate belong to the soul : they are transmitted to a denser body for a divine purpose."

[2] *Christ in You.* Published by John H. Watkins, London.

A brief consideration must now be given to emotion and its projection.

Anxiety is composite, ultimately it may be thought of as a compound of two opposites. The first of these is an emotion experienced as the natural positive reaction to danger, an affect which, for lack of a better term we may call life-hunger. The second is the reflection of another person's displeasure, probably mixed with natural animal fear. Both emotions are referred within, whence the riving of the psyche, a picture of which is well conveyed by Dr. Jung's expressive couple, the Will for Life and for Death.

At the merely animal stage there is a well-defined line of demarcation between the I and the Not-I; at this level the Not-I is eternally outside the I. Not so in self-consciousness, at which stage the reciprocal habits of Introjection and Projection potentially bring into the I (the self) everything within the entire range of experience. The dream shows this. There is nothing too remote or too insignificant to furnish dream elements and in the dream everything is the dreamer. Here there is no Not-I; the man we fight with in the dream is part of the dreamer equally with the object of solicitude and affection; sea, sky or mountain equally with flying machine or battleship. The human psyche is literally a microcosm as the ancients were well aware. In the dream a man can as well identify himself with a tea-pot or a flat iron as with angel, animal or devil.

But always we have to ask ourselves what do

these things represent and always we come back to the fact that all dream symbols exist to express an interior life with complicated organisation.

The stuff that this life is created from is energy, for which the only name we have is " emotion." Emotion is, roughly speaking, infinitely varied in quality, positive and negative, and further, since the sparking of anxiety is variously deep in different subjects, the emotional life of conceptual subjects must be of every degree of intensity.

All manifestations of emotion that are commonly seen do not by any means necessarily bear a constant relation to the stimulus in the situation; intense anger may be evinced as easily over a trifle as over a serious hindrance—that will depend on the subject. The emotional content of an experience, other things being equal, will depend, not on the stimulus but on the unconscious, or infantile anxiety situations which are tapped by the stimulus. The " other things," which are never by any means equal, represent the control of the subject, and this depends in great part on training, in part also, probably, on organic factors.

The finer differences attendant on the projection of emotion cannot well be understood until the Anxiety Drama has been dealt with. The discussion of the projection of emotion in this chapter must therefore be of a quite general nature; it will chiefly concern itself with the two main emotional determinants—life-hunger and anger-fear.

The first component of anxiety—life-hunger—is manifestly one with the interests of self. On the or-

ganic level it is "selfishness." In a panic men have
been known to trample the weak and to draw their
knives in order to cut a path through the obstruct-
ing bodies of their fellows.   We have no words
strong enough to deprecate selfishness, and yet we
know that selfishness is the *fundamentum* of life.
In the psychological sphere, selfishness is what
gravitation is in the solar system; it is the organis-
ing principle, without which there would be no
cohesion.   Everything would be perpetually out of
place.   Selfishness, therefore, must have positive
uses and, indeed, we find that it is the projection of
the unfathomable urge for self-expression inherent
in life.   In the poet's picturesque fancy God is
conceived as having created this world with all its
wealth of life that He might have objects to love
and to be loved by.   In smaller measure this is
what every human friendship aims at, no matter
how apparently misplaced the affection or how
incongruous the lovers. [1] It could almost be
asserted that the ultimate function of life on this
globe is to create a universal love-life; to expand
the self to include others, always probably through
some one chosen focus, star-like.   The more the
self-love, the more the raw material at hand for
projection.   A child's self-satisfaction, therefore, is
not to be despised—it is his conceptual stock-in-
trade, the fund upon which he may later draw vast
cheques representing amity and philanthropy.   The
educator's art is not to quench self-love, but to
direct its projection and to give it a worthy con-

[1] See Appendix I, No. 3.

tent. Far from being disheartened, let the conceptual subject who suspects himself of what he fears
is self-complacency remind himself that he is the
Life-Principle become self-conscious; that within
him is the Divine Spark; that, while his exterior and
physical qualities all reflect it, these are only effects
dependent on the apparatus and perishable; they
are not to be confounded with the reality springing
from an inner unseen source out of which the
unseen self is fashioned and by which it is peren-
nially sustained. This source is God, and it is to
God that he must direct his thoughts; so far as his
fellows are concerned, it is his chief task to create a
world where he and they together become one in
Him.

In their treatment of emotion, the older school of
Dream Psychologists appear to think that the only
formative emotional energy is that derived from the
sexual instinct. Dr. Jung, it is true, propounded a
theory of the *Hormé* (a concept very like that of the
Life-Principle), but he has, I understand, aban-
doned this and the higher functions of the psyche
appear in his system as they do in Prof. Freud's as
sublimated sex energy. I venture to think that
this misconception arises from the fact that sexuality as a dream symbol commonly figures most
insistently,[1] and that these schools overlook the
fact that in any case sexuality is only a symbol.
That sexual symbols do figure so persistently is,
however, partly due to the method of interpretation

[1] Providing the " romance " element which is so characteristic
of the dream. See Part II, Chapt. 2.

of these psychologists, for, as said at the end of the last chapter, insistence on a sexual and, in general, biological interpretation of the dream leads the subject to dwell on these matters and thereby rules the introjection process. If you begin by calling every sexual symbol in the dream " sex " and sex only, the subject's mind dwells on sex and his future dreams will reflect this preoccupation more and more, the further the process is carried. I do not find myself that the dreamer who studies his inner life on the Anxiety Hypothesis tends to dream so insistently of sex; rather is the contrary true. The dreamer becomes much more eclectic and general interests frequently furnish the major portion of the symbolism. The truth is that the Life Prin- ciple in all its manifestations is creative—not through the mechanism of sexuality only but through all its mechanisms. The Life-Principle is always building—bodies, groups, ideas, ideals. It is always progressive and inventive—*Creator*, not only *genitor*, is an appropriate epithet of the Life- Principle.

The second and opposite determinant in Anxiety is probably a compound of negative emotions— fear, hate, disgust, etc. We are familiar with negative emotions in the study of the instincts. Reference may be made, for instance, to the valuable hand-book by Prof. McDougall, called " Social Psychology." Leaving the dream study on one side, this book is an admirable description within a small compass of the development of human character. But to leave the dream out of character

F

study is to have the play of Hamlet without the character of Hamlet, as the saying is.

Negative affects as such do not belong to the perfected conceptual subject, they are in the first instance presumably incidental to the manifestations of the Life-Principle at the perceptual Level. Fear, hate, disgust are elicited in connection with the pain and deprivation attendant on organic experience. We must, however, assume that these emotions perform the incalculable service of cooperating in the sparking of individual self-consciousness when introjected as images before the projection process becomes stabilised. In the Anxiety Drama negative affects are directed against the untamed elements in the self which would, like Lucifer, assert themselves in opposition to that essential something in the self which we project as the Divine Will, and which I have elsewhere called the I-Not-I. As in the case of his self love, therefore, so in regard to his capacity, for aversion,[1] the subject need not deplore it. In it he may see the possibilities he possesses for victory over his own lower nature. Without this capacity crude elements of appetite could not be redeemed; he uses it for purposes of self-discipline. [2]

In the acting out of the Anxiety Drama the negative affects will be seen to suffer eliminations; they are reduced presumably to energy no less divine, but of an aspect presenting a contrast to that which we recognised as Power.

[1] Aversion is the opposite of appetite.
[2] See under Appendix I, No. 4.

We do our subject a great wrong, I imagine, if we allow him to abreact, *i.e.*, to project blindly, his negative emotions in excess. A certain amount of abreaction is probably necessary to relieve the strain of tension. The balance must be kept between the two lines which dream analysis should take, the first being association giving, the second the subjective interpretation of the dream picture. Dream associations always carry us back to significant and often painful episodes in actual experience. With these there will at once light up the emotions anger, hate, fear, jealousy, disgust, suspicion, which will direct themselves against other persons; also remorse and shame, the last two being more particularly anxiety affects and as such they are directed against the self, where as a matter of fact all emotions in the dream belong. The last fact becomes apparent directly the dreamer masters the idea that all symbols in the dream apply to himself. The effect of association giving is always to produce an eccentric action of emotion, whereas the effect of interpreting the dream as a picture of the self is to produce an opposite action of the emotions, a centripetal as opposed to a centrifugal or eccentric action. If we may think of the mute in violin playing as throwing the vibrations into the instrument we should have a figure of the action on the emotional life produced by the second phase of dream analysis! The first phase produces a loud noise heard by other people, the second, intenser vibrations within. As the second phase gains on the first, the insight of the student advances and he becomes master of his own emotional life to the relief of his fancied wrongs and his self-inflicted torments. But to accomplish this he must learn to regard himself as a spectator of the passions, which, with experience of the past, he introjected. I am jealous, bad-tempered, easily intimidated, but this is " not a bit of the real me " is what he will learn to say; he is learning to " think-in."

The Anxiety Hypothesis bases itself on the fact that there are two aspects of the Life principle, Power and Surrender, and that these are the component determinants of anxiety, moulding man's self-conscious functioning. These two aspects of the Life principle are no less to be observed in all manifestations of life, even at those most remote from the human. They come to light in the vegetable kingdom. We are accustomed to dwell on the power side of plant life—its colour, form and wonderful adaptive mechanisms, and are too much in the habit of applying sensory pleasure and pain as the criteria of happiness or misery. Hence, we forget that on account of relative immobility the vegetable kingdom is put under the ruthless domination of the animals which trample and rend it and appropriate its beautiful harvest of leaf and fruit without compunction.[1]

The law, universal in organic nature, by which one kingdom or one species makes prey of another presents a perfect picture of the second aspect of life—sacrifice, surrender. See again in what pro-

[1] *Cf.* George Macdonald's phrase : " Nature's endless sacrifice," and see Appendix I, No. 5.

fusion the lower organic forms have to bring forth their kind in order to ensure survival, with the inevitable result that, for instance, the pollen of some species powders the soil like snow, and the precious germs of forest giants perish prematurely in their millions. Is there no sacrifice entailed in the nocturnal habits of fierce beasts of prey or in the birth pangs of viviparous species? To recognise such facts of the interior aspect of life we must assume, of course, that the Life-Principle is one and indivisible, and in place of *cause and effect,* which are concepts furnished by processes of reason, we must set down *purpose,* the one-word equivalent borrowed from the terminology of the subjective aspect of thought. *Purpose* embraces the end from the beginning.

We can no more believe that the psychology of man, the most highly developed offspring of the Life-Principle on this globe, can exceed that of its source, than we can assent to the proposition that water may rise above its own level. We must therefore perforce allow that even in the vegetable kingdom the capacities of creative energy are rather dormant than absent, limited by apparatus provided for functioning rather than shorn of essential qualities. Life is the same life everywhere. On this globe, which seems a veritable school of adversity, self expression is everywhere balanced by surrender. Debit and credit tally on all hands; income and output in all directions tend to an equilibrium.[1] The very fact of the uniformity which

---

[1] See Appendix I, No. 6.

law involves proclaims the principle of self-limita-
tion.   Indecision in choosing a line of conduct is
at the bottom of much failure and misery in conscious human life, where obedience to law seems to
some extent a matter of individual choice.   The
offender is by no means always the sufferer.   Man,
alone, of all created beings, presumes in certain
crises to formulate the idea that dominion may be
divorced from responsibility and profit from loss, in
spite of the fact that his experience negatives with
insistence the possibility of such a contingency.
The lesson enforced by experience is entirely in the
opposite sense.   Pain-ceptors seem to multiply out
of all proportion to the capacity for pleasure, sorrow
to exceed joy.   This eternal discrepancy, it may be,
furnishes, in part at least, the data upon which man
founds his conviction that the postulated equilibrium demands a field wider than the span of human
life, individual or collective, whence the doctrine
known as the Theodicy or the Justice of God.

Justice we feel must ultimately transcend all codes
of human invention.   Human justice too often mis-
carries, and it is felt that adjustment or justifica-
tion of the balance is required, a function ascribable
to none inferior to Him Who is Himself the Life.
This is a common pivot about which all religions
revolve.[1]

---

[1] When a subject with irrational repetition complains that
people or things *are not fair*, he is expressing the fact that the
two aspects of his vital energy do not effect a balance.

PART II

THE ANXIETY DRAMA

CHAPTER I

SOURCES AND GENERAL CHARACTER.

And I said, moreover,
Haply what thou hast heard, O soul, was
Not the sound of winds,
Nor dream of raging storm, nor sea-hawk's flapping wings, nor
    harsh screams,
Nor vocalism of sun-bright Italy,
Nor German organ majestic, nor vast
Concourse of voices, nor layers of harmonies,
Nor strophes of husbands and wives, nor sound of marching
    soldiers,
Nor flute, nor harps, nor the bugle calls of camps,
But, to a new rhythmus fitted for thee,
Poems, bridging the way from Life to Death,
Vaguely wafted on night air, uncaught, unwritten,
Which let us go forth in the bold day and write.
              (*Proud Music of the Storm*, Walt. Whitman.)

In contriving the mechanisms of organic life, Nature, so prodigal in many respects, appears to favour the principle of economy. In the evolution of organic bodies, ideas are plentiful, but mechanisms few; rarely are old forms ruthlessly scrapped; new ideas and purposes generally mould new forms from older ones, the later arising through modifications of and additions to the earlier. No less does the principle of economy rule in the evolution of psychological structures and mechanisms.

It is the purpose of this Second Part of the present work to show the high purpose to which are put those apparently aimless experiences of early human life in which the subject, perforce, passively acquiesces, since motor co-ordination and language are not as yet his. In spite of the warnings of certain great educationists, well summed up in the saying imputed to the Jesuits, " give me a child until he is seven . . ." the usual view, tacitly assumed, if not openly expressed, is that, from the mere welter of baby experiences, the human psyche will arise phoenix-like to man's estate. In the process of education of the usual school age, it is assumed that the developing mind, above a certain standard, will slough the impressions of the earlier period, however brutalising and inconsistent, as some animals do the skin of the previous season.

While the warning of the educationist is undoubtedly justified, it is nevertheless the fact that something hitherto unexplained must underlie the optimism of general opinion. Why, it may be asked, is the man or woman born and bred in sordid care, perhaps even the sport of cruelty and vice, to be held in adulthood equally responsible with the man or woman cradled in comparative luxury and surrounded, at the formative stage, with every educational device ? Assuredly, a theory suggestive of the *tabula rasa,* such as Part I of this little treatise has presented, is not consonent with the common attitude to the problem of individual responsibility which has framed laws for and guided the moral destiny of nations. It is true that the Introjection-

Projection theory propounded in Part I does suggest that the conceptual aspect of the mind is at first a *tabula rasa*, but the difficulties which are incidental to this theory appear to be solved by the subsequent history of the material, introjected in as haphazard a way as trusses of hay are flung from all sides into the farmer's wagon. As the trusses are caught and set in place by the expert farmer's assistant, so no less the material introjected into the baby's mind undergoes a process of organisation, in conformity with principles of development which are here called the Anxiety Drama.

From a welter of ill-assorted mental images representing experiences of every degree and kind of variability, this process converts the introjected material into a harmonious whole presenting an average uniformity amid considerable diversity. The uniformity must rest, in the first instance, on the fact that physical instinctive interests furnish the bulk of the bottom layer of the symbolism. I contend that it is the organised presentation of introjected material in mental pictures which bridges the gulf between the isolation of the perceptual or animal level of the human psyche and the normal human mind capable of all that is involved by Professor McDougall's conception of active sympathy. In the process of harmonisation and organisation, which is normally one ending only with life itself, Introjection and Projection are necessary adjuncts and the action of these is not confined to *presented* experience only, but applies equally to *re-presented* material, *i.e.*, material presented as *ideas* detached from actual objects. Every fresh acquisition of knowledge, every further advance in the initiation into tradition, as into familiarity with topics of current interest, every book read, every lecture attended leaves a mark on the total product. This is why the educationist may entertain such high hopes, and, again, it provides an explanation of his apprehensions. Indeed, the part played by suggestion, which is almost another name for Introjection, can hardly be over-estimated. Apart from the group-life, what becomes of the future conceptual subject? and what is the evolved conceptual subject apart from the group? The group is, in fact, so much the Greater Self that the dream psychologist is particularly impressed with the responsibility of the adult generation in regard to its youth in general, and to its infants in particular. Yet he knows that the problem of personal responsibility will be shouldered by these latter in their turn, the explanation being that the introjected material, however unlikely, will arrange itself in the old familiar fashion, and, within certain limits of variability which we recognise as those of sanity, the new individual will be capable of coming into line with the common conscience and with the accepted attitude to the majority of human problems.

A fact never to be lost sight of is that the conception of the *tabula rasa* applies only to the conceptual aspect of the human mind. From the perceptual or animal aspect, the subject, of course, brings along with him a host of inherited tendencies. At the same time it is extremely likely that much which present-day teaching assigns to heredity is not really such.   If introjection play the part it seems, to judge from the dream, that it does, the child may well take over from parents and guardians both mental and physical habits.   If the child is in contact with timid persons, or persons of any other particularly marked disposition, it is extremely likely that his own character will reflect this.   Again, if a parent or any other relative has suffered from any particular disease, we shall expect it to reappear in the subject, or, at any rate, in his psychology. There are, it is true, what are called *reaction* formations to be reckoned with : the child in contact with a fussy person may, for instance, develop marked *sang-froid,* and so on.

What part genuine heredity may play in the process of conceptual evolution, apart from the fixed nature of the mass of symbolism which is derived from the life-functions—nutrition, breathing, sex, etc.—the dream psychologist has little means of judging.

I cannot accept Dr. Jung's theory of archetypes, as I understand it.   The semi-human, semi-animal forms which he classes under this name seem to be capable of a far simpler explanation.   They have all the appearance of perceptual tendencies which have been subjected to the conceptualising process in part only, and if an out-of-the-way animal is chosen to express this it is probably because the juvenile subject has been impressed by the sight of this particular animal at the Zoological Gardens or by the description of it and tales about it in his Boys'

Annual.   Analysis would surely unearth an association of this kind with comparative ease.

The mental images reflecting angry and pleased
faces and of painful and pleasurable situations introjected during and after the sparking process are
at first conceived by the child as having no reference
except to himself.   The impression that they are
within himself is the explanation of the special function of the dream, which is to transmute energy
from the perceptual to the conceptual level.   It is
because the first mental images are conceived by
the child as part of himself that they arouse him
from his " animal lethargy " and induce in him the
higher habits of thought.   The images must appear
as if occupying what can only be compared to a
stage where a puppet show is presented to which his
attention is *nolens volens* directed.   Again and
again the same image may arise spontaneously
under the influence of stimuli of a certain quality
and, creating new motor paths, they project themselves in early attempts at play, with, or possibly
without, the assistance of suggestion from the
grown-ups.   Certain features of the child's play
present what is practically a constant.   Where, for
instance, is the child who does not desire to take to
bed with him some article, often a disreputable, bat-
tered, ill-furnished doll or less recognisable article,
such as an old shawl wrapped up bundle-wise,
which he may call by a fancy name, a name often
reminiscent of some despised object or person?
This object is, of course, the self, probably, in the
expiation aspect.

A knowledge of simple language comes at the same time as play, and all the time new situations arise providing the material for further introjection. Sympathetic co-operation adds to the number of pleasurable pictures, and again, misunderstandings between the little subject and his guardians swell the bulk of unpleasurable images. By this process the framework of a self concept is constructed. Projection and again Introjection prepare the sketchy semblances of what will later be other concepts. From playing with the object which immediately represents the self, the child gradually includes other persons and their activities in his play; father reading, mother dressing, nurse sweeping, etc.—all concepts are derived ultimately from the same source as, and in terms of, the self concept, through projection of the latter. Thus is the waking anxiety life inaugurated, but by the very act of its inauguration a partition of experience takes place. On the side of Projection, the anxiety life normally frames more and more energetically, as time goes on, interests and purposes for the waking life, while, in the remote recesses of the inner consciousness, the original source thereof shrinks back into what is known only through the dream life. That the process of Projection is beset with difficulties has from one aspect been explained in Part I, and more particularly in Chapter VI of Part I. But there are difficulties of another kind incidental to the problem of the partition of experience and these consist in a confusion between the dream presentation and the experience of waking life. A story was told me recently of a little girl of five, which suggests to what a perplexing extent this confusion may hold. She was unusually absorbed and depressed one day during breakfast, and when pressed to say what the cause was, she said reproachfully to her brother, four years older than herself : " It was nasty of you to put that great big spider on me ! " The allusion was really to a dream and not to waking experience. The story suggests the probability of dream experience literally taking its place alongside of waking experience at a stage before the habit of Projection is thoroughly stabilised. This probably accounts for the many stories recounted of children with a tendency to " romancing " or " untruthfulness," as it is variously described. An example of romancing is that of a small boy of five or six, an only child, who for a short time entertained the theory that he possessed a little sister.

The dream life contains images of personalities which are roughly classified, in the present work and in the *Psychology of Self-Consciousness,* under two heads, namely Power and Expiation. But this crude classification gives the barest idea of that subtle interweaving of motives from which arises the host of conceptual emotions familiar to the human mind : joy and sorrow, repentance and resentment, shame and conceit, hope and despair, etc., etc. Mr. Shand has given a subtle and interesting analysis of some of these in *Foundations of Character;* Professor McDougall attempts to account for them all by compounding the well-recognised emotions common to human and animal psychology.

However we name them, these emotional entities must be conceived as referring in the original germ of the conceptual psyche—known through the dream life—to aspects of the self and the self only. Attaching originally to situations which were unmistakably favourable or unfavourable to the infant subject, they present an opposition in character, and between them the clash of conflict is soon discernible. In the midst of the conflict is the subject, at certain stages passive and not infrequently bewildered. When the dreamer says that something which happened in the dream surprised him, we have an important gloss on the dream. Power images and Expiation images are like two political parties between which stands the subject, like an inexperienced, or perhaps inherently weak, ruler—like Rehoboam, son of Solomon, between the older counsellors of his father and the young men who were brought up with him.

A dream cycle includes the shuffling and rearrangement of these two parties in surprising variety. Every dream subject has his own style of composition : some are expansive and detailed, others are singularly condensed ; now there are commonplace images and again imagery full of beauty ; some express themselves mainly through sensory images, others more particularly in thought. But, however different in treatment, the dream always has the same function : it is the guardian of an inner attitude to experience of some higher category, to something popularly called Conscience ; it provides a subtle index of the effects thereon of actual happenings. More than this, the dream cycle always has the same tendency; it develops the details of the method by which man proposes to make the great surrender of the toys provided for his conceptual training in this life.

Haply what thou hast heard, O Soul, was not the sound of winds,
Nor dream of raging storm . . .
. . . But, to a new rhythmus fitted for thee,
Poems bridging the way from Life to Death . . .

To these highly organised series of moving pictures the name Anxiety Drama seems most appropriate, for they reproduce all the features which we are accustomed to associate with a theatrical performance, as the following pages will attempt to show.

CHAPTER II

THE ANXIETY DRAMA APPEARS TO BE MOULDED BY THE SEXUALITY FUNCTION

Dream of a death, you hear of a wedding.
(*Proverbial saying*)

WHILE every external interest furnishes material for the Anxiety Drama, it is the bodily functions which symbolise the heart of the mystery, and among the bodily functions, sex, it would seem, holds the position of determinating factor. Indeed, the Anxiety Drama appears in the main to follow the scheme provided by the sex function. The sexuality symbol is to the dream what the iron frame is to the iron and cement building. That this is so we may conclude from the fact that the most obvious features of the dream, as well as its most mystic elements, derive their symbolism from sex; in other words, sex factors provide the *terminus a quo* and the *terminus ad quem* of the dream work, its *alpha* and its *omega*. In the first place the two main determinants are expressed by man and woman respectively. However absurd it may seem to the modern mind, the man is, for the child, the symbol of the positive aspect of functioning and the woman of the negative aspect, in spite of the fact that the child must be more familiar in general with the activities of the mother. In dream psychology, the

G

man *does,* the woman *suffers.*[1]   Every genuinely
selfish motive of a conceptual complexion *tends* to
be expressed as a male personality ; every genuinely
unselfish motive, on the other hand, *tends* to be
represented by a female personality.   It is necessary to say *tends* because the rule is by no means
invariable ; a dream personality represents, it
must be remembered, for the individual dream-subject his own particular reactions to a given person in
actual experience, and this fact may override the
general principle.   The dream of a sister strangling
a female dream-subject probably illustrates this
broader kind of treatment.   The sister *may* not
mean here the expiation or suffering possibility of
the dreamer in the act of subduing her, but
emotional experience provoked by association with
the sister in the original infantile situation.   In
instances like the above, the dream-moulder would,
in a general way, be at pains to transform the sister
into a male personality, someone, for instance,
closely associated with the sister.

The following dream provides a typical instance
illustrating the way in which the dream subject, in
analysing   emotional   tendencies,   makes   the
definitely egotistic ones masculine and the more
altruistic ones feminine.   " Miss G., Miss R. and I
had come by train to some station, bound for some
destination.   There is a man at the station whom I
had heard of before.   I think Miss G. knew him a
little.   He called a carriage for us and began put-

[1] Is it in thought relations of this kind that we may postulate
a hereditary factor in the conceptual sphere ?

ting us and some other women into it. I did not like this, and Miss R. and I began to walk away. The man, who was tall, slim and aristocratic in appearance, seemed to come with us and talk to us. Then he took us into a house and I was still more uneasy. After a little while I escaped from the house, leaving Miss R. behind. Then I was worried about her and I tried to get help. One man to whom I applied for assistance, who seemed like a butcher, would not talk to me at first; he seemed to suspect me. Then I thought of going to the police and I think I did so. It seemed that the man—a baronet, I think—was a man with a bad reputation."

The slim tall man of aristocratic appearance, who is afterwards discovered to be a baronet, appears on analysis to represent the subject's so-called " superiority-inferiority complex." From reading books of a sentimental kind the subject had early conceived the notion that the tastes of her family were distressfully plebeian and she longed for a more refined circle, one preferably with a scholastic atmosphere. The attitude of mind of the subject is plainly egotistical; the butcher's assistant is easily recognised as a sadistic element. Miss G. and Miss R., on the other hand, represent respectively the subject's willingness to perform domestic duties and her interest in sick folk. These latter are in danger through the " selfish " aspirations of the subject. [1]

[1] The subtlety of the above dream is remarkable. Miss G. and Miss R., as said above, stand for interest in domestic affairs and for suffering fellow creatures respectively. Note that the former is said *perhaps to know the abductor a little, i.e.,* in her

The above dream has an interest beyond that immediately under discussion. It also illustrates the subordination to the dream purpose of symbolism derived from the sex life, *i.e.*, the dream presentation has a preference for a romance setting.[1] It presents, on the lines of a sexual adventure, the doings of personalities which stand for anxiety interests, the dreamer expressing her apprehension about the fate of female personalities, her altruistic tendencies, under the figure of an attempted abduction. This is an interesting illustration of the generally constructive suggestiveness of the sexuality symbol. What the subject really fears is that a selfish purpose has rendered inactive, perhaps killed out, her genuine conceptual tendencies represented by housewife and sick nurse.

The main theme of the Anxiety Drama lends itself very particularly to the intricacies of the sex life, sexuality being in the symbol, death or self-giving, whence may arise the popular notion that dreams go by contraries.[2] Power misused is in general self-

interest in the home the subject's activities had been in part directed towards making it as beautiful as she conceived it should be. Note also that at the start the subject's social ambitions aimed at putting the women into a carriage, *i.e.*, provided a means of " getting on," which, in fact, it did, for it promoted a desire to pursue her studies, but that finally it confined them, shut them up in the house, *i.e.*, reduced her to a sedentary, creature-loving mode of life, while that which Miss R. stands for remained as a torturing doubt.

[1] By *romance* is here intended that mixture of love and adventure which is characteristic of the poems of chivalry produced in the Middle Ages by the European culture which arose on the ruins of Roman domination.

[2] See the proverbial saying quoted at the beginning of this chapter. Another well-known piece of evidence is the fact that Creator and Destroyer are associated as attributes of the same God.

love.   Self-love is "death" because love is destined
to be *projected,* such being one of the main purposes of the introjection-projection mechanism provided for the conceptual subject's training.   The
outward and visible sign of self-love is obviously
the giving of pleasure by the self to the self, *i.e.,* in
the sex life, masturbation.   Not greatly inferior to
this is any sexual gratification which does not entail
marital and parental responsibility ; the great symbol of expiation, therefore, is marriage.   Marriage,
in fine, is the favourite consummation of the Anxiety
Drama ; it is total surrender—" death."   All illicit
forms of passion are *death unto death;* sexuality
satisfied in proper moderation within the marriage
bond, by nature intended for the procreation of new
life (the child) is *death unto life,* the child symbolising rebirth—the genesis of the soul.   It is because
sexuality is associated in the symbolism with death
that all fear it, and consequently either abstain,
indulge with a sense of shame (conceptual fear), or
seek it in excess—the last because in the inner consciousness there is a restless sense of " death "
being deserved on account of infantile misdoings.

The sex drive in the woman can be no less than it
is in the man, but in general the woman is sexually
colder because she fears the passive side of the symbol which it falls to her share to meet in the sex act.
Hence the woman fears sexuality in all its guises
both in and out of marriage, and hence again she is
in general " purer " than the man.   If the drive of
infantile guilt is too strong the woman goes out to
meet her fate and becomes a prostitute of a certain

type. Death is accepted in symbol by the woman in the marriage act, the male organ symbolising the sacrificial knife. The man is the priest sacrificing the victim, the woman, as his substitute. It is the symbolism of the sex life which has invested man with priestly functions and made him the " head of the woman."

The man, on the other hand, is often sexually restless; he is driven by the sense of infantile guilt to seek many victims to suffer for him. Nevertheless, in his case as in that of the prostitute, because no love or service or responsibility accompanies the act, he is left not only not satisfied but with his debit account mounting up. Consequently, the more victims he has the more he wants. One reason why the sexually cold or impotent man may fear coitus is therefore because he conceives it as comparable in the symbol to murder; possibly in some cases he regards his expiation self, for which the female partner stands, in a light so ideal that it seems to him a desecration to approach her. In common parlance, the wife is the " better half." Sometimes the man exaggerates the sacrifice he is called upon to make.

In marriage, if one or other partner be unwilling for a child to be born, the other may become cold, because, strictly speaking, as said above, the sex act is only effectually redeemed from being death unto death in the symbol, *i.e.,* for the inner consciousness, by the promise of the new life, the child. The child is the self reborn. Let us suppose a couple marry and have children. So far so good. The symbol of unification is satisfied; power and expiation blend in the re-birth. But, conceptually speaking, the new life must follow. Love must be mutual, it must be uplifting, *i.e.,* it must concern itself with the higher values; the conceptual subject requires to have that from the lover which trains the soul for an after life. Love implies little attentions; it demands that which costs time as well as money; it is expressed by what involves effort and personal service. Every soul is seeking salvation and the lover is the saviour. If love which has once been given is withdrawn, a mortal wound is inflicted on the other partner because he or she has regarded the first as the saviour. Jealousy, strictly speaking, is the expression of the pain attending this mortal wound. The apparent withdrawal of love does not, however, necessarily involve the fact that love has turned cold. The case of the male (or " power ") partner who holds his wife in the light of a superior being has already been mentioned. More generally the apparent withdrawal of love is due to the unearthing of buried anxiety by some traumatic experience, like bereavement or reverse of fortune. Let the lover be slow to regard the withdrawal of love as due to a change of heart, for love once given is rarely withdrawn. But love is easily inhibited by fear or jealousy.

The married person who would be happy and make the partner happy should study the meaning and bearings of the great symbol which, by the fact of entering on the married state, he has advanced to the first rank among those symbols which will affect

not only his own life but that of others. The conceptual subject, realising that it is love which he is
really seeking, will be cautious how he plays with
a double-edged weapon. Sexuality may be called
double-edged because, as already explained, it
stands both for life and for death. If sexuality does
not satisfy appetite and quicken the subject conceptually, it creates appetite and ultimately destroys.
The desirability of exercising control in sexuality
applies not only where overt acts are concerned, but
in thought also. The undesirability of preoccupation with sex appears from the dream to have a
psycho-physical basis. By over-indulgence, physical
energy is kept in the lower centres of the cerebro-
spinal system—" downstairs," says the dream
language. " Downstairs " is a very apt description, for the nervous system consists of different
levels, which may well be compared to the different
storeys of a house. Energy in the lower centres
(or " downstairs ") is associated in the dream with
bodily disorders and aberrations of instinct. Pious
books written for the young on the subject of sex
undoubtedly reflect the fear of sexuality which
attaches to it in the unconscious.

All the above becomes obvious from the dream,
and there is no dream analyst of the impartial scien-
tific brotherhood who would or could deny in the
main the ruling of Professor Freud on the subject
of sexuality symbols in the dream. The importance
of the sexuality symbol is undoubtedly paramount.
Professor Freud has also shown beyond disproof

that the ambivalent attitude—love and hate—to father and mother is the ground of the dream work. The error is that he takes all these symbols, sex, father, mother, literally, whereby sexuality remains for him the sex function, in spite of all that may be said about it. The Oedipus fable taken by Professor Freud as a paradigm is again treated by him literally, though put back into infancy. In reality the tragedy of Oedipus Rex exhibits the subject in a crisis of the Anxiety Drama; the dream subject having slain his major power symbol, the father, and having merged his being with that of his major expiation symbol, the mother. Oedipus Rex must not be detached from all that is told us about Oedipus. Oedipus is a typical anxiety subject. The name Oedipus, swollen foot, suggests power subject. His exposure in infancy may perhaps be understood to correspond with the amnesia; his upbringing remote from home with the latency period, which means that as a consequence of normal preoccupation with the symbol in early life, he loses touch, as normally happens, with the inner anxiety self. He is just a jolly, out-of-doors boy, in fact father and mother are not known to him, i.e., niceties about power and expiation do not trouble him. The warning of Apollo, by which we may perhaps understand education, excites anxiety; he slays his father (? self-pleasing); so far so good; but the marriage with his mother—the real expiation situation—is precipitated by the reading of the riddle of the Sphinx.

The story of Oedipus cannot be detached from

this central episode. To read the riddle of the
Sphinx is to be brought face to face with the fact
of the shortness and apparent futility of human life.
It precipitates an anxiety crisis, the rebirth, perhaps, of adolescence. Success and kingship follow
for many years; Oedipus begets children, symbols
of the soul. In Oedipus Rex, a title suggested by
the irony of tragedy, we see our anxiety subject
approaching old age, faced with the anxiety problem in a new and urgent aspect, and as a result
he puts out his eyes and goes mad. This
self-mutilation may symbolise the withdrawal of
the psyche in old age and senile irritability. It is
the counterpart of Shakespeare's " sans eyes, sans
teeth . . sans everything "; it recalls the
psalmist's warning about the " threescore years and
ten, and though men be so strong that they come to
fourscore years, yet is their strength then but labour
and sorrow, so soon passeth it away and we are
gone." The trauma which precipitates the death
of Oedipus is the feud between his sons.[1]

The tragic history of Oedipus appears absolutely
in line with all wisdom teaching about the anxiety
career. The riddle of the Sphinx is a variant for
the " wood " in poems of chivalry and in fairy
tales; it is fear of death and of old age, the approach
to death. That which goes first on four legs, then
on two and finally on three is Man. He is first the
crawling babe, then the independent, erect, self-
directive being and finally the shuffling dotard.
" All men are mortal " is literally the first univer-

---

[1] See *Œdipus in Colonos*.

sal positive judgment which the human mind formulates when it reflects.

Oedipus slays his father ; in this is implied the general truth that, averages being taken, a curve would show that succeeding generations have risen to levels higher than those reached by the generations preceding them.   There has been a steady weeding out of savagery and barbarism, as self-consciousness has revealed them for what they are.This has been partly in consciousness, but it has also proceeded in the deep unconscious by a process of transmutation of energy.   It is not jealousy against the earthly parent which is intended by the Oedipus myth.   The bard is chronicling after the manner of his kind the rise of the divine sap in the human tree.

Oedipus marries his mother, so complementing the overthrow of the father.   Man not only achieves a conquest over the lower and selfish impulses but he goes a step farther and embraces self-sacrifice. The embrace is fruitful ; noble aspirations of the more virile sort (sons) and also of the more sacrificial kind (daughters) are born, aspirations of the soul and doughty and charitable deeds on this plane.

The neurotic is one who has slain power, but along with power in its undesirable forms he has lost his capacity for normal practical functioning. Every anxiety subject must complement the slaying of power by embracing a life enhanced spiritually by a better understanding of the problems of suffering and duty and by a cultivating of that divine knight-errantry which goes forth cheerfully to the encounter with all and everything that may betide. This spirit of service and resignation it is for which in these latter days the Messianic or Christos symbol is universally accepted—symbol expressing the fact that man is learning to bear the everyday burdens of the flesh in his own person instead of pushing them on to the shoulders of beasts, slaves and women, and others, for him, outcast—symbol of the fact that by the very bearing of these burdens man is raised and not lowered—raised indeed to sonship with the divine, made the heir to individual immortality. Man does not become God. He becomes inalienably merged in Him, while retaining his own individuality.

Interpreted on these general anxiety lines, the story of Oedipus exhibits a human soul between the two anxiety determinants, Power or life-hunger and Expiation or surrender. For the purposes of presentation, the story is cast in the mould of *romance*. This, as has been explained, is what is done in the dream quoted at the beginning of the present chapter, where a story of abduction is selected for the treatment of material remote from real sexuality; the same is true of the Oedipus story. It is the romance form of presentation which never grows old ! Schools of artists and thinkers have over and over again arisen in the past, cultivating different methods for presentation of wisdom teaching,[1] but always the youth of the world returns to romance. Anxiety literature, in the main, follows the line of

[1] See Part II, Chap. 4. Variants for the Romance Form of the Anxiety Drama.

the dream.   Love is the " old, old story," because the bi-sexual subject, between his two determinants, is for ever striving by self-conquest to achieve unification, and by projecting love to create a conceptual universe.

The Oedipus story is like many a dream in the handling of the affect.   The horror of the story supposedly attaches to murder of the father and marriage with the mother.   Really it arises from the anxiety which underlies the hero's quickened reflection on the problems of existence.   The displacement of the affect in the dream has been described by Prof. Freud.   A study of this topic is absolutely necessary for the understanding of dreams.   Probably it is the setting of the dream which is the displacing agent.   In the Oedipus, as so often happens in dreams, the setting has the *romance* character.[1]

[1] The ancient tragedies are said to have been written originally by *adepts* for the instruction of *initiates* in the *mysteries* of human life.

CHAPTER III

THE PLOT IS COMPLICATED BY THE SUBJECT'S REVOLT

Men must work and women must weep.
(*The Three Fishers*, Charles Kingsley)

THE little child objects to the restriction of his activities, and equally he resents exclusion from favour. He brings no criterion of right and wrong along with him from his animal forbears. Life is life for him until the parents supply the criteria for the selection of preoccupations. To eat so long as a thing tastes good, to snatch a coveted object and appropriate it for his own satisfaction, to find interest in matters relating to his own body and its functions, these are as natural and desirable from the child's point of view as breathing. But precious energy required for the conceptual life must not be too recklessly wasted along these lines. If no solicitous parent be at hand to inculcate the rules of decency, the child's group, in its own interests, will not long tolerate asocial conduct; the subject will be ostracised. In these circumstances, habits which are undesirable, if persisted in, will have to be indulged surreptitiously. Here is one source of danger; another is, that the child may rebel vehemently. Unless he understands the reasons for coming into line with the social conscience, a child will become an outlaw or indulge in secret. In either case he becomes a law unto himself.   The child may be full of subterfuges, for, though he bring no moral code with him, he is the embodiment of intelligence, that " filler in of gaps," as Professor Hobhouse says, wherever the instinctive process is menaced with failure.   If Mother has put the coveted foodstuff on a high shelf in the cupboard, there are, at any rate, chairs and tables which may lend themselves as a means of reaching it.   The child, therefore, tends, in the first instance, to function as power subject, and it is as power subject that the dream supposedly first presents the subject. Nevertheless, the opposite "party " formed out of introjected material of the opposite quality, is somewhere in the immediate neighbourhood, and its relation to the power " party " supplies the anxiety drama with an infinite variety of situations.   That the infantile mind is the scene of many a conflict, for which it probably gets no credit, is plainly seen both from dreams of the immediate period and from dreams of adulthood, which frequently contain infantile material.   Possibly, if properly handled, dreams of the infantile period would be of great assistance in the child's training.   The dreams of childhood show a great deal of mental tension.   A small boy dreams that a giant comes with a sword and threatens to cut his head off.   The violence of the crisis is evident.

The undisputed dominance of the power party does not, as a rule, last; the juvenile subject is warned early.   This, it seems, is the intention of the above dream, as it evidently also is of a dream in which the devil is cutting the subject's nails. The devil is unmistakably regarded as an evil agent, the giant is just the power sense. The difference, probably, reflects the attitude of the respective parents to the delinquencies of their children. Cutting off any part, commonly described as *castration* by dream psychologists, is an infantile form of expiation. Possibly the child is at first anxious about any interference with nails and hair, and may bring nails and hair-cutting into line with care of the teeth, any interference with which is a typical and dreaded expiation situation even in adulthood.

Simplicity is a marked feature of infantile dreams, but the child-dream, it is necessary to say, is no more a simple presentation of a wish fulfilment than an adult's is. I should entirely disagree with Professor Freud on the interpretation of infantile dreams. The dinner that disappears cannot be understood as having been eaten. Cooked foodstuffs are commonly used by subjects interested in culinary processes to represent the mind or soul under discipline. The following dream illustrates well the treatment of this symbol. The subject had cooked some potatoes, but thought there were not enough, so decided to cook more. This she did, putting them in with a pudding that she was cooking. She was very pleased with the result; the potatoes turned out well—" nice and floury." The subject, on the occasion she recited the dream, had begun the conversation by remarking that the rather difficult situation in which she was placed was relieved because she had put more restraint on

her reactions than formerly.   She expressed the
opinion that, with persistence in this attitude of
mind, her difficulties would be overcome.   She was
altogether more mistress of herself than she had
been before; in fact, she was in what might be described as a " chastened mood," but there was also
cheerfulness observable.   Discipline situations projected are described popularly in just this language
of the kitchen, as witness, for instance, " in a stew,"
" in the soup," " in hot water," etc.

On the other hand, the little boy's dream of a
plate of cherries, all of which he ate, is susceptible
of a very subtle explanation. It obviously reflects a
temptation situation; it is with situations of this
kind that fruit is commonly associated; the classic
example is the story of the Garden of Eden.   There
is much more in the cherry dream than a mere wish
fulfilment associated with indulgence of the
nutrition appetite.   The child is more than a mere
repressed animal who has " made up " or imagined
a way of consoling himself for deprivation.
Imagination is a word relating to the highest faculty
of the human mind; it has been seriously debased
through a deeply rooted habit we have of imputing
inferior motives to ourselves and others because we
have forgotten the symbolic efficacy of everyday
experience and the titanic conflicts of childhood.[1]

To analyse the dream elements : *Fruit* is that product of the plant which contains the precious germ

---

[1] Also the modern psychologist does not discriminate phantasy
from other more legitimate functions of the imagination. See
infra, pages 167–170, for a discussion of the phantasy habit.

of future life. It always stands in the dream for
forbidden knowledge. The other element, *eating*,
" I ate them," is equivalent to " making experience
of," " taking-in," as we say. All taking-in of
human knowledge, whether secular or divine, is, in
the symbolism, eating. Some knowledge, like
some food eaten, is nutritious, some unsuitable,
some again positively poisonous. The unsuitable
is inherently associated with the nutritious, and the
discussion and ventilation (evacuation) of this
unassimilable part is a necessary aspect of the subject's training, hence the insistent part played in
dreams by the defœcation act. " I was looking for
a lavatory," " I was on a lavatory seat," or " passing a motion," somewhere inappropriate, etc., are
common elements in dreams. The extrusion of
unsuitable material leads to a sense of being " relieved " or " purified," whence the euphemisms,
" lavatory " and " water closet." To revert to
the cherry dream, I conjecture that the meaning
of this, taken comprehensively, is that the
subject has been either having experience which is
prohibited, or receiving information about a forbidden subject. The dream so interpreted constitutes, in fact, a variant of the Eden story.

The Eden story portrays the situation in the
Anxiety Drama which may be called the *revolt*.
Every child who lives to man's estate, has come
through, what Dr. Jung calls, " coercion to domestication," and has been in the Eden situation. It
is a situation which the genuine psycho-neurotic
has never forgotten, perhaps even he may never

have left it. As the child cannot get his way by direct means, indirect methods for achieving the same present themselves; they are the fruit borne by the tree of the knowledge of good and evil. What a conspicuous object of the garden is that tree! How attractive its fruit! How delicious the flavour in anticipation! Dream subjects tell the most sympathetic stories of early conflicts with the arch enemy, self-pleasure, stories in which we catch glimpses both of " spoiling " by parents and its opposite. In their love, the parents dwell on every feature of their beloved baby, and, contrary to expectation, baby knows a good deal about it. In the dawning of self-consciousness, can the child fail to be impressed with its own charms, considering the attention paid to them? Equally certain, the child insufficiently appreciated by the grownups, will find preoccupation with the self-attractive, but he will cherish the cult of the self in secret. The child sees the reflection of himself in the mirror and he is impressed with the daintiness of the picture, the freshness of the colouring and the harmony of the moulding. But self-love is deprecated. Then there appears on the scene a personality whose subtlety is greater than that of all other beasts of the field—the serpent. " Yea, *hath* God said? " asks the revolt subject, " can it be that the beloved Ego must be subjected to prohibitions, be made into a servant? Can there be another who compares with the I ? " And the subject turns with surprised pain from some significant discipline situation, or from the newcomer, baby brother or baby sister, with whom the eulogies and tender demonstrations erstwhile his alone must now be shared.

Driven back into self-love, the subject asks again, " Yea, *hath* God said ? " But the God-principle, primitively within, has by this time spoken, to the little subject's chagrin. He knows, moreover, his utter helplessness in face of it. This is an experience typified by the awareness of nakedness, a typical dream element which frequently, in some form, in the actual dream analysis, gives the first indication of dawning self-knowledge. " They hid themselves, for they knew that they were naked."

Conceptual insight may have first arisen in, or at any rate, been first expressed by, male subjects reduced to slavery, into whose cortical cells fierce nervous energy, set going by bitter physical conditions accompanying limited opportunities for self-expression, may have introjected an image of the tyrant's queen. Eve is possibly a real queen personality, herself a budding conceptual subject, beloved of the dreamer whose dream has furnished the Eden story. In the dream she represents his feminine self in revolt. Despite the curious conceptual phenomenon, which we know as misogyny, the conceptual subject is destined to be in love with his introjected expiation symbol through its association with the new life, and with this symbol, the human mind has eternally associated woman. As a result of revolt, the guilty pair are expelled from Paradise, *i.e.*, from innocence or guiltlessness, but the promise has been repeated from gen-

eration to generation, that in spite of all
sin, sorrow suffering and shame—" though he (the
serpent) shall bruise thy heel, thy seed (thy soul
symbol) shall bruise his head." But the immediate state of the pair is one of toil for him and
suffering and dependence for her, and the way of
the tree of life is barred by an angel with a flaming
sword.

This slight picture is limned with the singular
accuracy of the dream work; it furnishes a compre-
hensive view of all the various ways in which the
conceptual subject symbolises his means of salvation (which are, at the same time, his penitential
offerings), grouped under three heads :

1. There is first the sexuality symbol, the labour
and anguish entailed by subjection to the great
principle of death and re-birth. It has been treated
at some length in the last chapter. " In sorrow
shalt thou bring forth children and thy desire shall
be to thy husband," is the curse pronounced on
Eve, the female personality of the conceptual (bi-
sexual) subject.

2. Man's activities, represented by the working
of the soil—the curse pronounced on Adam—are,
as a matter of fact, seen constantly in the dream
linked up with the expiation theme. Experience
of the material difficulties of existence and mastery
over material resources, have become associated for
man in a very special way with his inheritance of
suffering. It has come about that, as introjected
material, the objects wrought by hand and brain
become beautiful because they represent, often, the

specific disease, which is at once a symbol of the sin to be punished, and the means of atonement. Instances of the dream treatment of this theme will be given in a later chapter. In passing, we may notice how the association has infinitely enriched human culture, for it imports symbolic efficacy into every labour of hand and brain. The power subject may scamp his tasks and attempt to commute his liabilities into a money payment, but the expiation subject never. Consequently, it is suffering which mixes the artist's paints, which lights the seven lamps of architecture and which inspires not only soldier, sailor, and adventurer, but the devotees of such humbler tasks as gardening, carpentry, penmanship, needlework, cooking and housewifery, generally.[1] Suffering, the *leitmotif* of the expiation subject, prompts a man to carry out exquisitely the details of that which as power subject he projected grandiosely. We are one and all, in the unconscious, in love with death—the way of retreat from the school of life—so soon as we find out the illusoriness of a brief power phase. Does man reserve his worst imprecations for two opposites, the suicide and the murderer, because the first curtails the term of initiation into the mysteries of suffering and the latter deprives a fellow man of the chance of fulfilling his?

The flaming sword — disease — bars equally for Power and Expiation subject the way of return

---

[1] The Christos principle is to be detected under the image of any common workman in the dream. Cf. *Piers the Ploughman* and the woodman in *Red Riding Hood*.

to Life. It is surprising how the old symbolism holds the human mind. In an advertisement, recently displayed everywhere, asking the charity of the public for London Hospitals, the fire-symbol recurs. Instead of flaming sword, however, the angel had *wings* of flame. Flame still bars the way for the infantile revolt-subject to the Land of Promise, in spite of all the advances in medical science. As a symbol of disease, specifically, fire holds the first place in dream symbolism.

The revolt subject, as I have said, appears in the Eden story as the serpent. The serpent is the embodiment of subtlety, he is " worldly knowledge." The study of the dream acquaints us with the aspect of the subject who is the counterpart of the serpent. He will not discontinue asking, " Hath God said ? " He comes to the fore under various dream figures. I recognise him, for instance, in a dreamer who is playing cards for a stake of £5, with a woman in white. In this particular dream, the subject dreams that he loses.

Jesus links up the Messianic title, Son of Man, with the serpent, in a way which has special significance for the dream student. He says, " As Moses lifted up the serpent in the wilderness, so also must the Son of Man be lifted up." Moses did, according to Numbers xii, 9, make the semblance in brass of a serpent and expose it to the view of the Children of Israel when they were attacked by serpents and— this is most important—*those who looked upon the symbol were healed.* As a dream analyst, I endorse the fact that the subject who will—or rather, who can—look at his own expiation process, i.e., the serpent lifted up, in the Anxiety Drama, in a way sufficiently objective, gives the best promise of rapid rehabilitation.

" Son of God " (the other and greater Messianic title), as I need merely indicate, is the successful conceptual subject—the subject who merges happily from the purification of his microcosm, a process completed by the lifting-up of the serpent in the wilderness. Perhaps a variant of the lifting-up of the serpent is the symbol familiar to mysticism of the serpent biting its own tail. This introduces us to the immense subject of the great conceptual affect, remorse. The serpent biting its own tail forms itself into a mystic symbol of immortality, eternity, infinity. This is the same as the " ring " in the dream—the ring, emblem of marriage, and of the victor's crown.

CHAPTER IV

THE EXPIATION PHASE OF THE ANXIETY DRAMA

A heart alone
Is such a stone,
As nothing but
Thy power doth cut.
(*The Altar*, George Herbert)

ON the Anxiety Hypothesis the final phase of the Anxiety Drama is recognised to be Expiation. The end anticipated is of a tragic character, presumably because the end of existence on this globe is for one and all death, and for self-consciousness this fact is ever present somewhere in the mind. The end anticipated is always tragic, but equally certainly the dream subject seems to anticipate that when the curtain is rung down on this side of the veil there will be as surely a raising of the curtain which admits to life elsewhere. While there remains a reckoning, a day of account—for every child of man is a revolt subject—there is always something after which the dream subject in some obscure way is groping, an expected evolution of some kind which is supremely desirable—something for which all the pains and penalties of this existence are well worth while.

Professor Freud has observed the frequent recurrence of the examination dream; he observes that the *finale* of this dream is generally expected to be that the subject fails to satisfy the examiner. His comment on this dream is to the effect that the dreamer, having been a successful competitor in his examinations, hereby expresses fear on account of sexual impotence, but couples with it the wish to be no less successful as a lover than he was as an examinee. *The insufficiency of this explanation*— right, so far as it goes, for impotence, is a negative attitude to the power determinant—is easily detected by the Anxiety Hypothesis. The same latent content belongs to dreams in which the policeman intervenes, or the subject finds himself in a court of justice. The examiner, the policeman, and the judge, vary according to the material introjected, and their rôles are infinitely various because the revolt subject is of every degree, *i.e.,* the sense of sin is greater or less in everyone.

The need to balance power with expiation is observable in the psychology of even little children, as the following incident, brought to my notice by a teacher, exemplifies. In a class where little children under five years old were busy upon the modelling of plasticine objects, a small boy of two years and ten months was making a steam-boat. It had a famous funnel emitting a quantity of smoke, and on the hull of the ship, which was conspicuously small, was an object which resembled a cross. The teacher asked the child what this last object was, and he replied to her surprise, with something of reproach in his voice : " Jesus ! " She pressed for a further explanation, and he said, " Jesus stilling the waves." So the small conceptual subject,

under three years of age, fashioning a power symbol, adds a cruciform figure to the composition for
balance !

It is necessary, in introducing dreams of the expiation phase, to emphasise the fact that the part
played by *actual* bodily suffering to-day is in great
part a misdirection of energy, due to the materialistic attitude of the modern world to anxiety problems.   The subject would treat much which works
out as disease far more successfully if a sound psychological attitude were inculcated.   The body is
only symbol, and the task before the conceptual
subject is *not* to project suffering on the body *but to
effect a balance*.

The interests of expiation, in competition with
power, are handled with infinite variety by dream
subjects   and   the   same   dreamer's   attitude   at
different stages of his career is shown by the introspection   process   to   have   been   conspicuously
different.   The two following dreams illustrate the
difference of attitude   of   the   same   dreamer   at
different times.   In the first dream the subject is
going up a hill and turns to look at the view.   *It is
a scene in the downs; the land slopes down from her
feet to the valley and rises on the other side.   Not
far below her is a wild rose in perfect leaf, but the
flowers have all given place to the most beautiful
berries.   There are many sprays all laden with
haws.   She exclaims with delight.*   From my
knowledge of the dream work, I feel confidence in
saying that this wild rose, laden with haws, represents a physical condition for which the dream sub-

ject has twice been operated on, the second time quite recently. Her expression of delight is tantamount to an attitude of acceptance of suffering and gives evidence of the fact that a promise of harmonisation between the conscious and unconscious levels has resulted from a comparatively short psychological re-education. The same subject's earlier attitude to the expiation phase is expressed in the following dream which she brought almost immediately after the one related above. *She is walking along the esplanade of a seaside town and sees two advertising bills lying so crumpled by the wind that she cannot make out in full the words on them, which she knows announce a series of religious services. Afterwards, her mother insists that she shall attend some religious services. She reluctantly consents, and, to carry out her project, proceeds down some disagreeable grey-looking steps and finds herself in the basement department of a shop where she is to buy a clergyman's outfit. She has a pattern suit with her which is very worn.* The religious services are the operations and correspond, in general, to the same complex as the wild rose bush covered with berries of the earlier dream. The change of affect in the dream, *i.e.*, the change of attitude towards the expiation phase in the second of these two dreams, reflects most faithfully the change which accompanies the bringing of the subject's dream-life into the crucible of the Anxiety Hypothesis in consciousness. Whereas she had previously felt hopelessness and aversion in regard to life in general and to her immediate circumstances in particular, she is now looking at life almost with cheerfulness, and certainly with expectation. Yet her outward circumstances are not different, the change consists in a recognition of the fact that her attitude to the problems of suffering and discipline in early life were hopelessly at variance with the general tenor of her feelings in relation to the same problems in the deeper layer. Here, in the unconscious, the severity of her upbringing, introjected, was providing an affect entirely opposite to the manner of working of the same factors in the waking life. When these different systems are seen in juxtaposition the Dream mentor is satisfied and the dream can proceed to its appropriate *finale,* apart from projection on the body.

Indeed, when the nature of the anxiety problem is really understood, the subject of average intelligence and good mental organisation accepts the facts with hearty acquiescence and can afford to smile even while still suffering from a certain amount of depression arising out of the past conflict. The results on the unconscious of such a subject are equally remarkable. Sullen indifference and gloomy foreboding give way to acceptance of the facts so gladly as to advance the symbol of suffering and punishment into a thing of artistic value. It becomes an object of adoration. All the most beautiful things are worked into the picture according to the taste of the subject; flowers and fruit, as above, carving, painting, needlework and ornaments of exquisite workmanship, have all appeared in the dreams of my subjects. When the subject has less insight the same objects may occur in the dream and the note of caressing admiration be absent. I give two dreams which illustrate this. The first is from a patient suffering from exophthalmic goitre. The goitre is represented in the dream as a piece of board wrapped round and round with fine muslin. It evidently stands for the body from an inert aspect, and it is located in that special part of the physical economy, because in the dream the neck and throat appear frequently as the *bridge*. The " bridge " is that which, in the symbolism of the body, connects the apparatus of the conceptual and perceptual subjects, respectively. The meaning is, that the infantile bodily preoccupations have been an obstruction in the development of a highly-organised, most amiable, and entirely well-meaning character. The second dream I give *in extenso. The dreamer has arrived at a bazaar where she is to act as saleswoman. She is looking at the articles which are to be sold, before the bazaar is open. The only article named is a dressing-table cover, worked in cross-stitch.* All affect is seemingly absent from this dream. The subject being new to the treatment and extremely reserved, I explain the dream without questioning her as to its import. Indeed, my conviction with regard to the latent content of dreams and the function of the dream as the transmuter of energy is so confirmed, that I feel no hesitation in giving an approximate interpretation. Later on, as she is able, the subject must fathom her own problems. I explain that the saleswoman at a bazaar is engaged in selling, not for personal gain but for an object certainly disinterested and possibly religious. The subject's attitude to the expiation phase should not, therefore, present any hindrance; it is, on the contrary, the guarantee of rehabilitation, if it can be made to harmonise with the waking consciousness. The cross-stitch I interpret as referring to an operation which she had had two or three years previously, shortly after losing a much-loved sister. I am convinced that the dream is the result of explaining to the subject the general principle that the dream is appealing to the subject to recall and think over previous experience which has not been properly assimilated and harmonised with the general trend of the yearnings of an anxiety subject. As a result of this interview, I think, the subject on the next occasion brought a dream with the following manifest content. *She and a married sister, seated together at a window, receive by the hand of a stranger, a man, a message from the deceased sister, about whom the two at the window had been feeling some apprehension. The letter directed the dreamer to come and fetch her sister at a certain place where there was a wood. The dreamer accordingly went and found her sister, contrary to expectation, quite happy, playing hide-and-seek with others of her party.* The dreamer felt some chagrin at having been troubled unnecessarily. The meaning of the dream is that the fear of death (the wood), introjected through experiences in connection with the illnesses and death of a delicate sister, specially beloved, was found to have fewer terrors for the dreamer than she had known. The affect, the chagrin, is, of course, displaced and may be inappropriately described.

Two points relating to dream interpretation are to be gathered from the above examples. In the first place, the direction taken by a dream analysis, which is working well, is from present-day experience to more remote experience. In this way the deeper problems of the unconscious are prepared for through adjustment of more recent aspects of the same problems. The dreams themselves constitute, in these circumstances, a sure guide. An analysis is not going well when the dreams present a medley of indeterminate fragments. This reflects the conflict of many levels aroused simultaneously by the very fact of bringing dreams up time after time and leaving them unsolved. The unsolved fragments bring a host of negative affects, hate, fear, suspicion, which invade consciousness in a riotous fashion. On the Anxiety Hypothesis these affects will melt before the rising luminary of the expiation determinant if the transference is good and the subject sincere. The subject *has* to learn to look upon the serpent lifted up in the wilderness scene of his own anxiety life, and whether he can do this depends to a large extent on seeing the Anxiety Drama in perspective. He has not leisure for this while he is abreacting his negative affects aimlessly in consciousness. At the same time much good is done by a certain amount of discussion of the subject's difficulties, doubts and sorrows, whether past or present. The analyst must, above all, not stand between the subject and his repentance, while holding the balance fairly between the genuine claims of the infantile sense of sin and the present-day consciousness, which either ridicules or is nauseated by phrases familiar to any form of confession, such, for instance, as " miserable sinner." The secret of success is for the subject to allow the Anxiety Drama to occupy as little as possible the stage of present-day consciousness. He must, as already said, relegate the conflict to the smaller and more remote stage, and the words of Aristotle, to the effect that the passions are " purged " by witnessing the representations of dramatic art, will prove particularly true here.[1] The objection felt by some people to theatre-going may express a projected fear that exactly the opposite of this will happen ; it is feared that this separation of experience will not take place, but will rather be hindered by witnessing dramatic performances and not be helped, as the Aristotelian principle claims. If these objectors are right, there must be something seriously wrong either with our dramatic art or with our preparation of the subject for life. If the importance of the drama were understood, it would be an object of the educationist to initiate the subject into an understanding of the relation be-

---

[1] The *Eumenides* of Æschylus are a foreshadowing of an enlightened psychological rehabilitation of the neurotic. The Furies (sense of infantile sin) are not banished but placated. They are assigned their place in the conceptual sphere. From curses (Dysmenides) they are converted into blessings (Eumenides). *Cf.* the promise that sorrow shall be turned into joy.

I

tween representations on the stage and the Anxiety
Drama in the recesses of his own inner consciousness. The same initiation mediates between the
subject and his religion, I find.

A second point to be noticed about the re-educa-
tional process is that normally the affect is
not released until the genuinely spiritual attitude
towards the problem is shared by unconscious
and conscious alike. Want of the habit of a
spiritual outlook in waking consciousness, is, therefore, a real hindrance to complete rehabilitation.
Without it, mere analysis does not tend to bring
about a spontaneous balance, but, on the contrary,
it tends to produce dissociation. Many subjects,
under analysis without constructive assistance,
resist dissociation to the bitter end, some being unwilling to let go the power determinant and others
refusing to entertain the expiation determinant in
any shape or form.

This is the secret of the apparent obstinacy of so
many subjects. An analysis which is devoted to
preoccupation with any symbolism, but especially
with sexuality, as an ultimate, only emphasises the
conflict and increases the breach between the two
determinants which it was intended to remedy.
Cases which have had the Freudian treatment are
very much more difficult to re-educate on the
Anxiety Hypothesis than cases which come
fresh to the new process, presumably because
this dissociation has reached a fairly advanced
stage.

There are two aspects of the Life Principle de-

scribed by students of religion; one the projected
concept, God, the other, the Life Principle become conscious in organic nature and self-conscious
in man.   The first is the Divine Transcendence,
the second the Divine Immanence.   In the great
religions the first is in general mainly before the
mind of the builders of those religions, the priestly
caste.   Of the two aspects of the Life Principle,
Power and Expiation, it is the first, the I AM,
which monotheistic religions hold up for adoration,
Jehovah, for instance, in Judaism, and God (or God
the Father), in Christianity.   Power would normally come first, as every subject first knows in
himself the I-Not-I, the constraining indwelling
power which militates against the selfish impulses.
In time, room is made for a second concept.   In
Christianity it is The Divine Son, the Soul principle
emerging through the action of the expiation determinant—the LAMB slain from the foundations of
the world.

The Christian Church has long authorised the
adoration of this second principle.   Though not,
perhaps, apostolic, the practice is extremely natural
and, from the point of view of human psychology,
as seen through the dream, it appears to be an inevitable evolution.

But what has become of the Divine Immanence
in religion?   In part it is represented by the care
bestowed by the priesthood on the worshipper's
soul, but this, with every fresh reformation in
religion, tends to fall more and more into neglect.
A difficulty seems always to have been felt with

regard to the Divine Immanence. In the history
of the Christian Church the difficulty has always
existed. It has been expressed sometimes by the
opposition between the mystic and the theist, and,
again, it has taken the form of controversies between exponents of the faith principle and exponents of the principle of intellect. The fundamental difference in these points of view, expressed
by the mysticism versus theism and faith versus
intellect, reflect *stages of the Anxiety Drama.*
Would not a study of the dream, that great transmuter of energy, help towards a reconciliation of
these differences? Many of our divisions may
merely be due to the fact that man does not know
his own nature. Dream psychology could supply
an education of the individual worshipper which
would fill the hiatus and make the doctrine of Immanence more intelligible and more stabilised for
the ordinary man without detracting from his
efforts to reach out after the transcendent God. The
two are really complementary and cannot be sep-
arated without prejudice to the anxiety life. To
understand the principles underlying the causes of
cleavage in human thought would be an incalculable boon. The cleavage creates untold confusion in the minds of the average person who cannot
see the necessity for hating those who take one side
or the other. There is so much of pressing practical importance in modern life that the average person already alluded to leaves the confused and con-
fusing controversies on one side through sheer
weariness and despair. I speak from bitter know-

ledge; an earnest search for truth may find the
seeker at the end of many years more puzzled than
at the beginning.

What has become of the cult of the Divine Immanence? Has it not been left mainly to all and
sundry—nursemaids, asylum attendants, police
officers and hospital staffs? In other words it has
been neglected quite unwarrantably. A study of
the Divine Immanence seems to be a thing for
which mankind to-day is thirsting. Attempts are
being made all round to supply the need.
Theosophy, Christian Science, Higher Thought,
are all such attempts. All have provided text-
books, but the primer has been wanting, and it may
prove that the study of the Dream on the Anxiety
Hypothesis is just this primer. If we take with
entire consistence the Freudian dicta that the dream
is symbolic and that its latent content presents a
unity, the transmuting capacity of the dream easily
becomes apparent to the observant dream student.
It may be that through the study of the dream every
human being with a capable and sincere guide shall
have it in his power to con the great primer of the
Divine Immanence. The true democrat, the phil-
anthropist, will take notice.

But the primer must include the whole subject,
not the emotions and the instinct life only, as Prof.
Freud very naturally assumed at the outset. Dream
symbolism shows that body, mind and soul are all
inextricably involved. So long as the primer falls
short of this, it is small wonder that many anxiety
subjects will continue to prefer to grope along their

own darkened paths than to submit to a process which may only lead to blacker darkness.

The significance of dreams can only be arrived at by the most patient co-operation between the analyst and his subject. The human mind cannot be dissected in anything like the way the organic tissues can. There must be give and take between two or more rational ethical subjects, and it is only as the subject of marked paranoiac tendencies is won over to rational and ethical insight that progress can be made. Until the secret of this transformation has been found the analyst must be the embodiment of patience.

CHAPTER V

VARIANTS FOR THE ROMANCE FORM OF THE ANXIETY DRAMA

I fled him down the labyrinthine ways
Of my own mind ; and in the midst of tears
I hid from him, and under running laughter,
　　Up vistaed hopes, I sped ;
　　And shot, precipitated,
Adown Titanic glooms of chasmèd fears.
　　　　　　(*The Hound of Heaven*, Francis Thompson)

As already explained, the common form of the Anxiety Drama is outlined by the sexuality symbol and a romance setting is the one favoured in the dream as it is in anxiety literature. The sexuality symbol is compared in Chapter III to the iron frame of an iron and concrete building ; however covered up, the great symbol is always embedded in the structure. But a sexuality theme does not always confront the observer; there are many interesting complications and even variants. " Labyrinthine ways " expresses perfectly the tortuous courses by which the revolt subject seeks to evade the climax of the Anxiety Drama. Some variants are serviceable, and being approved in group life, have apparently come to stay. Others have marks of disserviceability and are considered morally reprehensible. The group is not agreed in regard to certain others. It is impossible to treat schematically in a small compass so large a subject. I propose, therefore, to deal only with two or three of the commonest dream schemata which exhibit a deviation from the original—the normal sexuality symbol. The most important of these is the Christos concept, a picture of which is drawn by Francis Thompson, in " The Hound of Heaven," quoted at the head of this chapter. In the last chapter, I suggested that the Power concept, which every religion presents in the first place for worship, will be duly followed in the course of evolution by a second concept corresponding to the second determinant of anxiety. Many religions show this development as a masculine personality : Hercules, Prometheus, Buddha and Mithras, all express the idea, more or less, but in none is it worked out so simply and effectively as in the Christian religion. The Christos concept is an important variant for that of the Mother; at the same time, it is much more than the Mother concept, for it also embodies the concept of the self re-born. The Roman Church has, perhaps, been true to human psychology in allowing the concept of the suffering Mother to remain beside that of the Son.

The Christos concept may well claim the title of Mediator, for it spans many chasms and fills many breaches in human psychology. In the first place, it abrogates the difficulties of misogyny ; mediation is and has for a long time been sorely needed between the pride and independence of the individual power subject, on the one hand, and the despised, yet fear-inspiring, Mother image on the other. This is true to-day in the dreams of both male and

female subjects, and many social problems consequently find their solution in the Christos concept;
by it the dangers of "male passive homosexuality"
(to use Dr. Ferenczi's term), are decreased and provision made at the same time for the increasing
expansion of woman's individuality.

In this way the Christos concept mediates between the unconscious and conscious levels. In
general, it acts in the direction of transmuting the
mere interest in suffering into the joys of service.
Indeed the Christos concept lends itself exquisitely
to the needs of every forward-reaching soul. It
holds up a picture of self-love projected in its
entirety, a goal for the sense-conquering subject to
whom this life is yet interesting and joyous. It
presents us with that perfect blend of male and
female which any and every gospel of the conceptual life will increasingly furnish. The Jesus of
Christianity in every way invites the conceptual
subject's adoration. " Born of a Virgin," " made
of a woman," may be interpreted to signify *offspring of sheer suffering,* one whom an infantile
conception of power has touched but never
tarnished (" tempted in all things, yet without
sin "), one in whom the luminary of power shines
reflected altogether from a body of suffering and
surrender as the moon reflects as soft radiance the
brilliance of the sun.

As marriage is the projection of the drama at
the point of harmonisation of the two great determinants, so friendship is the projection favoured
by the subject who is unconsciously occupied with

the theme of the re-birth.   The sex object may often, conceptually speaking, be no more than a fear object, awakening anything from awe to hate, and that is why the child so often usurps the place of the married partner, and why a friendship may rank as high or higher than marriage. But friendship commonly awakens a certain fear as it seems to involve the shirking of the responsibilities of marriage.

Francis Thompson chronicles his flight from the tremendous Christos concept : Anxious nights and days are described in a few nervous phrases :

> " I said to dawn : Be sudden ; to eve : Be soon,
> With thy young skyey blossoms heap me over
> From this tremendous lover ! "

He relates his wooing of nature, and every touch reflects mental states now depressed and now exalted :

> " *I* drew the bolt of Nature's secrecies,
> *I* knew all the swift importings
> On the wilful face of skies ;
> I knew how the clouds arise,
> Spumèd of the wild sea-snortings ;
>   All that's born and dies,
> Rose and drooped with ; made them shapers
> Of mine own moods, or wailful or divine—
>   With them joyed and was bereaven."
>   etc., etc.

But the chase draws closer, all fails him :

> " Even the fantasies, in whose blossomy twist
> I swung the earth, a trinket, on my wrist."

In his anguish he cries :

> " Ah ! must thou char the wood ere thou canst
> Limn with it ? "

The majestic figure is in sight now :

> " With glooming robes purpureal, cypress-crowned."

Until reduced to :

> " A strange, piteous futile thing."

The poet surrenders to the summons :

> " Arise ! Clasp my hand and come."

Not every soul fascinated by the Christos concept is so recalcitrant. In the stories of the Quest of Holy Grail or Sangreal we have those who themselves *go in pursuit* of Him with the " glooming robes purpureal."

The poets, however, who treat this theme seem impressed by a certain coldness in it. In William Morris's poem, for instance, Sir Galahad is described, in the hour of despondency, as reflecting on the joy of those who are blessed with a mortal love, on the warm arms of Guinevere twined about the neck of Lancelot, and, as adding pathetically in reference to his own fate, " Ah ! poor chaste body ! " The Heavenly Master, however, speaks words of comfort :

> " Fear not
> You are uncared for, though
> No maiden moan
> About your empty tomb."

Mortal love receives the opposite of commendation, and of Lancelot, it is predicted that he, too, will have to earn salvation by coming to the feet of the supersensuous Christ :

> " For Lancelot,
> He in good time shall be my servant too.
> *   *   *   *   *   *
> Yes, old and shrivell'd he shall win my love."

Surrender, moulded on the Christos concept, is a feature in the dreams of many subjects. One of the most striking of these represents an eagle nailed to the Cross. Sometimes the dream replaces the last tragic scene of the Crucifixion with dream elements reminiscent of the Last Supper or the Agony in the Garden.

The Cross itself, or the Cruciform Church, often occurs as the symbol of the suffering body.

The Christos concept adds infinite dignity to human consciousness, raising even the meanest act of service into the Divine Life.

> " Who sweeps a room as for thy laws
> Makes that and the action fine."[1]

There is no outcast in Christianity.

When the love component of the self-concept has not sufficiently gained a way to projection, the difficulties in the pursuit of salvation loom large. We then meet in dream and story every possible expedient for staving off the expiation phase. Hence —as if the hands of the clock could be arrested—

---

[1] George Herbert.

" the child that will not grow up," the indolent, self-indulgent, tearful woman, or the irritable dependent man. It is pathetic to see the blend of pitiful dependence and arrogant self-assertion in others, and humiliating to detect it in oneself. And it is so often associated in the same subject with high courage in times which are really critical, the whole making a strangely inconsistent picture.

Where love is insufficiently projected, energy is apt to display itself as puerile " negative " in face of every trifling obstacle. It is this aspect of the expiation subject which dream psychologists of other schools confuse with the whole " Mother fixation." " The male is strength, the female weakness, man positive, woman negative," says an academically-trained young male subject, who has gathered his knowledge of the dream work mainly from the books of these authors. But this is not what the dream itself says; is this not a scrap of misogyny escaped from the dream level into the thinking consciousness of the authors? The dream, indeed, says rather the contrary, i.e., that the principle of self-giving is higher than the principle of self-assertion; perhaps more strictly it says just what modern biology teaches that both male (the sperm) and female (the germ), are equally necessary for the procreation of the new life. The subject, who approaches his dreams in the spirit of the youth quoted, will, in the long run, only add to the torture and conflict, although he may temporarily experience relief in the sphere of waking consciousness. If the Anxiety Drama act itself through, and the conscious subject merely assist as an interested and sympathetic spectator, it will be seen that through the staging of the expiation phase there is not permanent loss of anything of manliness or capacity for positive functioning, but that, on the contrary, only the puerile elements of power are purged away. Through disregarding the real import of the Mother as a dream image, many psychologists encourage in their subjects the very kind of character they deprecate. A subject, training on the Freudian principles particularly can easily become the incarnation of dependence, and at the same time develop an unlimited amount of " negative " to so-called " authority " in general, and to relatives and friends, and even the analyst in particular. I am pleased to observe that the teaching of the Anxiety Hypothesis definitely does *not* foster this particular infantilism, but, on the contrary, rather corrects the tendency if it has appeared and restores to the subject a genuine fairness of judgment which is the first criterion of sanity. To preserve the *balance* is the great object of the anxiety method. To damp down anxiety is naturally the first impulse of the conflicted soul, and among expedients for saving the self, the easy one of blaming another person for the predicament one is in, is not long in suggesting itself. Adam, in saying " The woman thou gavest me to be with me, she tempted me and I did eat," is the prototype of the subject who goes into ecstasies of hate, whether in relating his troubles to the psychologist or in the privacy of his own thoughts. It is slumbering negative which

often frightens the subject away from analysis, but
I do not think it should really be an obstacle.   It is
true that the passivity and ignorance of the subject
put him originally as a little child at a great dis-
advantage in the introjection process, and the negatives may be considerable, but to possess an ordinarily organised waking consciousness *now* is
proof that the conflict was never past remedy and
will not be unmanageable for the particular subject in the re-education process.   Subjects in states
of definite mental disorganisation may present a
different problem, but even for a subject who has
had to be put temporarily under the care of medical mental experts, the strain of re-education should
not be more than can be supported if the subject is
under proper instruction and has a sympathetic
friend to shelter him.   Meanwhile, it is evident
that if the subject has come through his troubles
and disappointments up to the time of treatment,
he must be capable of going back over the past and
by picking up the threads reorganise it.   It
must be painful, and it will take time; there are no
miracles done by the psychologist, as Dr. Jung
says, but it can be done if the subject will, and it is
worth while.

Among expedients for arresting anxiety, the use
of alcohol and drugs is a time-honoured one.   There
is everything in the worship of Dionysus from the
most beautiful to the most revolting, from the sweet
pathos of the lyricists to the stern tragedy of Euri-
pides.   In the *Bacchae,* Agave, under the influence
of the God, tears her own son limb from limb, be-

lieving him to be the sacrificial animal. Under the influence of the God, Dionysus, who takes away the fineness of waking perception and works confusion in the brain, the expiation phase goes forward to an accompaniment of wild delirium or blinding intoxication. If the final phase must come, the idea is that the brain must be either artificially stimulated to behold the apocalyptic vision or reduced to a dazed condition beyond the consciousness of happenings on the plane of sense.

There is but a step from the damping down of anxiety to that variant of the dream finale which is the subject of the Faustus story. " A short life and a merry one," is a proverbial saying still in the mouths of men and women ; there is a disposition in certain anxiety subjects to take any risks, to barter their hopes of salvation with all its possibilities, but with the certain tedium of its pursuit, for one moment of this life of which it may be said *Weile doch, du bist so schön* (" Tarry, I pray, thou art so fair.")

The story of Faustus is best known through Goethe's treatment. According to Goethe, Faust, the scholar, wandering gloomily in the fields, observes a black dog approaching by diminishing circles. It is Easter Day, and his attitude to the festival is shown by his comments, suggested by the sight of people walking about, which may be paraphrased thus : " Yes, it is the Resurrection, for is it not spring time when mankind arises from narrow streets and alleys and goes out once more into the glorious open under the sky ? "

For all his rationalistic interpretation of the Christian Festival of Easter, Faustus is a prey to superstition. The black dog which enters the house with him could only do so, he supposes, because the pentagram on the threshold is imperfectly drawn—Mephistopheles, the black dog metamorphosed, undertakes to introduce him to that supreme moment of which he has dreamt—but the payment is to be his soul. " The moment " involves the callous betrayal of the beautiful and innocent Gretchen, whose story is drawn by Goethe in a few situations, masterful in their pathos.[1]

Apart from the particular variant already described, the barter of the soul, the Faustus story introduces other features interesting from the point of view of dream psychology. We notice in the first place the inset moulded on a romance plan, the story of Gretchen. Gretchen is the feminine counterpart of Faustus, and the latter works her ruin and indirectly that of her child, his soul symbol. This, on examination, is seen to be a parallel to the main theme, the barter of the soul. It is one with the haunting *coitus* dream so familiar in the psychology of a type of male subject. One subject

---

[1] A drama which Lessing had projected, also dealing with the old Faustus legend, has an interesting development. From a letter of Engel we learn that Lessing intended that the terrible story of temptation, crime and punishment should prove a dream, angels having buried the real Faustus in a deep sleep to protect him from the plotting Satan, and replaced him by a phantom. On awaking, Faustus thanks Providence for his escape, and says he is now more possessed by virtue than ever before. This treatment of the story is a natural one in view of its truly terrible character.

K

says that he has had periods of dreaming of *coitus* with every woman he sees, and this obsession, obviously embodying a death wish to his own feminine self, marks an intense reaction against the expiation phase, which yet holds him so firmly that he identifies the feminine self with every woman seen.

Another notable element in the Faustus story is the scholarship of the hero. A love of scholarship must always owe its initiation to the revolt. Scholarship may be interpreted as an attempt to wrest a solution of the problem of the inner life and so avoid the appointed way of suffering; " to spend," as Clough says,

> " Uncounted years of pain
> Again, again, and yet again,
> In working out in heart and brain
> The problem of our being here."

Consequently, there is a kind of youth, who, in spite of undoubted capabilities, cannot succeed with his studies, for every step towards success is deprecated in the dream life and encounters a strong pull of the expiation call.

The idea of bartering, the main line in the Faustus story, is very prominent in much dream psychology and much of it has an application which is similar to that in the Faustus story. To buy sweets and dainties, for instance, or a special type of hat or boots or other clothing, may express a striving to retain sense experience, or, having it clandestinely, to look right in the sight of others, and the implication may be that the dream subject is willing to pay

in chances of salvation.   Paying is effected by giving something of standard value for the perishable
symbol.   Money, the lineal descent of faeces, may,
in general, be taken to represent what in religion is
known as " merit," and the explanation may be
that in the child's psychology the passing of a mass
of faeces is confused with child-bearing; in any case
it stands for the giving up of something precious
and private.   Almost every element in child psychology meets in the defaecation process.

Another variant suggested by fear of the expiation phase is that the subject is incapable of having
a soul, or being unable to emerge from a spell—
that of the lower nature—which confines him to
the level of beast or even tree—the latter a purely
vegetative existence.   Souls imprisoned thus, re-
quire, in order that they may be set free, the volun-
tary sacrifice of a Saviour or devoted maiden.   This
theme is a familiar one in fairy tales, *cf. Beauty
and the Beast, The Frog Prince,* etc.; dream
equivalents of this theme probably mark a deep
dissociation.   In theology its counterpart is an
attitude expectant of " Salvation through Grace ! "
The inner life is in a condition of stasis and some
intervention from outside is awaited.   Subjects of
this kind leave everything to the analyst and attri-
bute their failure to him if they do not understand
the situation.

The last variant for the romance form of the
Anxiety Drama, which may be mentioned in this
chapter, is drowning.   As Prof. Freud and his
school point out, this dream, which is fairly com-

mon, seems to contain a reference to childbirth and
the waters of parturition.   Their judgment is that
the dream is a mere fulfilment of a repressed wish
for physical motherhood. Really it brings together
in one symbol the idea of self-immolation (expiation) with that of the re-birth, and is an exact parallel of baptism, a sacrament of which the inner
meaning is, " a death unto sin and a new birth unto
righteousness."

PART III

THE SELF THROUGH THE DREAM

CHAPTER I

THE PROTAGONIST IN THE ANXIETY DRAMA AND HIS CONCERNS

> One hour, I believe, in that consecrated clinic (the Confessional), is likely to teach a priest more of the richness, the latent beauty, the truthfulness, the humble effort and the divine and lovely secrets of humanity, than even a year spent in contemplation of life's evident successes.
>
> *God and the Supernatural.*   Fr. Martindale, S.J.

THE conceptual subject is the protagonist in the Anxiety Drama, for, though he does not always appear in the drama, and although, if he appear, he does not by any means always take the principal *rôle,* yet it must be remembered that every one of the *dramatis personae* is part of himself and that he is always, in effect, the stage manager and directive agent. Whether he appear amid his own dream population or not, the affects apply to him in spite of all appearances to the contrary. An instance in point is a dream in which the father is represented as angry with his daughter, the dream-subject, whereas, of course, it is really she who is angry with him, because the father is dream image representing her own power.

The conceptual subject who has any degree of
insight and is, in consequence, what we call a sensitive or earnest person should welcome the fact that
in his dream life he may find guidance and inspiration. For in the waking life the average conceptual subject is, I think, very hardly circumstanced.
What earnest soul is there that cannot tell the story
of an anxious search in youth for some clue to the
problems of existence, a search which never came to
an end and was probably relinquished through dis-
couragement—" hope deferred."   The water of
life is everywhere, but it cannot always be drunk;
it is made bitter by many devices.   The very knowledge that should feed the soul is made unpalatable
or apportioned in such a way as to be unsatisfying;
the result, as often as not, is sheer starvation. One
subject is brought up on worldly wisdom—this is
like a diet of nothing but, let us say, carbohydrates;
another is reared in a circle where religious practices
are enforced *ad nauseam,* this we may compare
perhaps to a diet in which proteids are in excess.

Again it is true that "one man's meat is another's
poison," *i.e.,* symbol systems build barriers.
A man's own symbol becomes a panacea, it
crowds out others, and therefore impoverishes life
in relation to the one thing that is of supreme importance—sympathy.   The subject stakes everything on cherishing his own symbol, forgetting that
the symbol is, after all, perishable, whereas that for
which the symbol stands is imperishable, and that
here he and his brother subject may really find
themselves agreed.

We seem to be incapable of using experience in its true and natural proportions. We have not got what Jesus means by " the single eye."

The amazing fact which has been forced upon me in the course of my work with psycho-neurotics is that the bodies and souls of men and women are sick—sick often unto death—because the inner experience is presented to them in such a way that it robs " the universe of rationality," as a subject once put the matter in a voice in which was literally a ring of despair.[1] As a dream subject then, man demands a rational universe, strange inversion as this seems of what is universally held! The fact that after their first youth few appear to care in waking consciousness is nothing to the point. In the unconscious, every subject cares desperately; what people seem exteriorly is mainly a matter of group suggestion. The first thing the group demands, and *rightly demands,* is that the subject present a reasonably acquiescent attitude to social ideals; if he can be got to do this his educators are, in the main, satisfied. Immensely important as the discipline of the group life is, it can be forced too far. Where the strain of endeavouring to satisfy these ideals cannot be borne by the subject a physician is consulted! I must frankly confess that I regard this as an anti-climax. If mankind could not submit to a system of spiritual masters, is it going to submit tamely to the domination of masters who assess the needs of humanity

---

[1] What this subject may have had in mind is discussed below, pages 172 and 178.

from the most mechanical aspect? Kind and conscientious as the average physician is, it is staggering to one who has studied the inner life of dozens of subjects to hear the anguish of the precious human soul appraised in terms of bodily diseases and the remedy thereof in terms of patented medicines and operations.

In the dream, mental states are conveyed by images of the body, and states of disharmony depicted in morbid physical conditions, just as in the anxiety literature of the Hebrews the sin of Israel is compared to putrefying sores. On awakening, the thoughts of the subject turn on the dream images, and the subject feels impelled to consult his medical man. Will the conceptual subject never attain to the true vision of himself as a unity, and apply himself to learn what is the genuine nature of the innumerable ills that flesh is heir to, and the real method of release therefrom? Must we always be under the heel of some *one* profession in the community, which, through the sheer immensity of the task before it, tends to take the most mechanical view that can be entertained of the material in its charge? If the Church fail, will the medical profession succeed? The human being is one, and while the principle of economy suggests the removal by medical means of all hampering causes in respect to the more mechanical part of our make-up, and while religion—that great first projection of anxiety, must ever hold a place all its own in helping the psyche to *cosmosise* her cravings—something more is needed. This need is met by the intimate confessor and teacher, who will draw out, as the educator should, all the beauties and possibilities of the individual soul lore of which the quotation at the head of the chapter speaks so feelingly. Medicine, Religion and Psychology, should co-operate in the healing of man.

The function of Psychology is a very definite one. The dream is always calling upon the subject to harmonise experience. Something happens in present-day experience (the stimulus), which links itself up with that mass of undigested psychic experience which we call, collectively, the unconscious. The stimulus has a vitalising relation to this apparently waste material, which, in spite of appearances, is capable, according to the economical methods of the Life-Principle on this globe, of being fashioned into the means of working out for each one an attitude to past, present and future, which will produce harmony, beauty and happiness. The great possibilities of the dream have, for a long time, been a closed book to man because the dream was not understandable until the key to its code had been discovered (or re-discovered?). This discovery we owe mainly to Prof. Freud. But the principle of the symbolism of the dream must be rightly understood. As already explained, to take *any* part of the dream imagery at its face value decentralises energy, and this is bad for mind and body. We project energy along the lines of symbolism which figure in the mind as ultimates. Up to a point, as shown in Part I of this book, literal projection of the dream symbol, which operates all the time automatically, has a beneficent function, but beyond a point, or applied in a certain way, it has definitely bad consequences. The conditions we are now able to control, thanks to a consistent interpretation. To interpret dreams on the right lines acts in the direction of centralising energy. This process is beneficial for mind and body. It conserves energy. Every subject is found in the process of dream interpretation just at the point at which his education in this sense has been hindered, and on his own lines and at his own pace he moves forward in the direction of inner harmonisation. The beauty of the process is a surprising revelation.

The dream psychologist stands in wonder at what revelations may await the researcher. The reciprocal processes of introjection and projection display experience in two series, objective and subjective, which have a striking correspondence so far as the waking intelligence can follow them. All starts from the nuclear equation, body = mind. His body stands for the subject's mind, his house for his body, gardens and all beautiful and sacred objects, for his special application of the expiation principle to body or mind or both. Again, bodily functions represent mental processes; alimentation and elimination are figures of these processes which build up the inner life through the intake of experience and keep it wholesome through the ventilation of that which is indigestible. All voided experience, i.e., experience discussed, like the voided waste products of the body, becomes the fertilising soil or manure for another season's crop; breathing portrays the subtler relations of the psyche with the unseen sources of her being. Along the organic line the dream subject gives evidence of a much deeper comprehension of physiological facts than we have any idea of in waking life. He probably knows for instance an almost indefinite amount about the structure and organs of his body. Presumably the same intimate knowledge of purely psychic conditions is his, and when we get to know what, in their dreams, the more deeply sparked subjects are able to tell, much which is at present guess-work in waking consciousness, and hence properly called the hidden or occult, may be released from this category and become the common heritage of mankind.

It is because the two series, the objective and subjective, bear such a close relation or correspondence to one another, and because the symbol as projected is so aptly and exactly suited to the inner term of the comparison whenever the opportunity reveals it, that we are emboldened to believe the same correspondence to hold in relation to that which is at present beyond the ken of waking consciousness. But in most subjects there is a great gulf fixed between the subliminal consciousness and the waking consciousness. The dream apparatus which should bridge this gulf is, in our present state of knowledge, commonly a great hindrance instead of a means of communication, because the fears it contains act as a *vis a tergo,* keeping the attention on the symbol. The dream is full of fear because it is built up in infancy and it contains unassimilated anxiety experience of the most intense kind. The dream cycle presents itself as conflict between the Will for Life and the Will for Death and is, therefore, unintelligible to the waking consciousness which can only will life. To be " willing life " in consciousness and " willing death " in the unconscious, is to subject the psyche to considerable strain—strain which cannot be easily tolerated; nevertheless it is this condition of things which is regularly present in what has been called the " periods of strain "—notably in adolescence and at the climateric—and in many human lives periods of strain are recurrent because it is a condition of things stimulated by all waking experience which is of the nature of a shock. The psyche without assistance must therefore protect herself from the intrusive entry of shocks and her equipment in regard to this has been called by Prof. Freud the *resistance*. Resistance prevents the subject allowing the internal state of things, if at all one of order, to be disarranged, and consequently he makes himself impervious to suggestion. Suggestibility, as ordinarily understood, would seem to be a mark of the seeking psyche, the psyche in comparative dis-ease. The psyche whose affairs are comfortably settled will resist suggestion and interference, and this seemingly desirable state of things may result from two opposite conditions, one in which either the waking consciousness prevails or one in which the Anxiety Drama, or a special phase thereof, holds its own successfully and cannot be dispossessed. The deeper and the more dissociated the psychic trauma, the more impervious is the subject to the suggestion of his fellows. But as just said, the entrenched waking consciousness is also impervious to suggestion.

The subject with a high resistance, unable to tolerate introspection for the Anxiety Drama, is a painful revelation to this subject in the waking consciousness. Orienting his attention outwards, he has built up a wall between himself and it, not allowing stimuli to awaken the fears of the Threshold, but staving off anxiety by every conceivable device. So long as he can, he projects vehemently, grumbles and hates, works unreasonably hard, or perhaps is inordinately full of good works. When anxiety has heaped itself higher than he can dispose of by these methods, the remnant is generally expressed somatically. Then the subject comes into the doctor's hands. But if the psyche is bent upon staging the *finale,* no medicinal treatment will avail. Operation will follow operation, the disease will spread from one organ to another, or assume one metamorphosis after another—and the doctors will shake their heads and say " we cannot do impossibilities." In rarer cases the energy escapes as abnormal conduct and the sufferer is then classed as insane or criminal, according to circumstances.

It may seem to many inadvisable to disturb the psychic equilibrium in the case of subjects who externally present a psychic picture which at all approaches the normal, but the psychological re-educationist, even in these favourable circum-

stances, may not agree with this judgment. From
the dream it would appear that human life on this
globe has larger issues at stake than mere comfort.
Human life in the present phase may be compared
to a boarding school. The primary object in both
cases is not to be happy at any cost, but to be
educated, to put in effort—" to scorn delights and
live laborious days." At the same time just as it
is important that the life of a child at school should
be happy, so it is important that life on this globe
should be reasonably happy, or the energy available for tasks will be dissipated. Extremes are
what it is desirable to avoid. It is possible for the
subject to be too absorbed in the problems of the
present, as this may lead him to regard all concerns
beyond those of the immediate present as an intrusion; equally, the subject must not always be
pining for another condition, for that will not profit
himself or anyone else. The object is that he shall
live—here while he is here, but always with a view
to the larger life which flows around the present
material plane as the ocean round an island—at
least such in the dream subject's view. It is analogous to the cosmic outlook of science, which is
its projection—an outlook reaching into unfathomable *subjective* deeps, as the *objective* outlook
reaches into innumerable world systems.

In the circumstances of confusion in which the
conceptual subject of to-day finds himself, it is not
surprising that humour has reached such a development. As Prof. Freud has pointed out, wit and
humour contain covert allusions to the sexuality

preoccupations of the unconscious. And the explanation is enriched when we reflect that sexuality is the greatest symbol of the conceptual subject and that the inner meaning of this symbol is in the first place death, and only secondarily life—life through death. In laughter there is courage in the face of this, courage expressing itself in every degree from the depreciation of obstacles which might temporarily stay the forward-reaching impulse in youth, to the great stand made by the soul watching its own agony in the supreme hour. And there may be bitterness, too—bitterness expressing " I would not, but I must," bitterness with a keener edge expressing " rather you than I," and the supreme bitterness which is at bottom a curse.

It is the element of incongruity, it is said, which provokes laughter. True, but the *apparent incongruity, the laboured manifest content which we call " the joke," is only a shadow of the great incongruity*: We ask life, and what is presented to us is, in the first place, death.

Laughter and tears, in fine, are twin expressions of self pity. Tears are often shed where laughter is anticipated, and laughter heard where tears are to be looked for. Psychology teaches how much these anxiety reactions are a matter of habit and training, and hence inculcates respect for the extremes of both. I never realised how nearly akin these apparently opposite anxiety reactions are as I once did when I heard in a public place a sudden sound which I took for loud weeping. It was uttered by an adolescent girl. On turning, I saw

the young subject to all appearances laughing.
Why is laughter tolerated when we could not
tolerate tears? Is it the increment of courage
which commends it? The reverse of course also
holds, for in the ears of some, perhaps of all in some
moods, laughter reverberates intensely painfully.
Truly has the Wise Man said:

" There is a time to weep and a time to laugh."

The incongruity, which is always an element in
wit and humour, is, however, nothing else fundamentally than tragic irony. The story of Oedipus
which, in Chapter II of Part II, was analysed on
anxiety lines, illustrates perfectly what in connection with the old dramatists is known as tragic
irony. The hero, even while expressing confidence in his security, is yet seen by the spectator
to be rushing on his doom. Oedipus, warned by
the oracle, and intending to safeguard himself,
flees from safety to the scene of his doom, and later
he insists on the introduction of the very witnesses
who will reveal that he is the slayer of father and
incestuous partner of mother, the father of sons and
daughters who are also his brothers and sisters, that
hence he is himself the man for whose iniquity the
land is plague-stricken.

Life to-day is as full of tragic irony as were the
dramas of Greece. The power subject by night
dreams of escape or of salvation under figures which
by day work his ruin! The murderer, the miser,
the gambler, the drunkard, the wife beater are vic-

tims of the conflict between their power-urge [1] and the symbol of expiation. The expiation subject admires most rapturously that symbol which in the dream figures the devastating disease.

We aspire to autonomy; we must therefore enquire into, and control, the psychological mechanisms which will render us autonomous, otherwise we are like the child clamouring for edged tools and explosives, before having learned the A.B.C. of their purpose.

In waking consciousness, what the conceptual subject must before all things aim at is to maintain the *balance* which represents sanity. Sanity and health are balance. When the subject tends to feel unduly elated or depressed he must remind himself that action and reaction are equal in the emotional life as truly as they are in problems involving physical forces. To maintain a proper balance in waking consciousness and to direct attention to some interest, no matter what, so long as it is useful and elevating, and so to maintain self-control, will help to banish the Anxiety Drama to that inner stage where it belongs. Here it may with great advantage work itself through with intelligent psychological assistance, so producing the desired unification of character.

[1] The power-urge is not the simple perceptual craving as so many of my critics appear to think. See " An Answer to Some Criticisms " at the beginning of the book.

L

CHAPTER II

THE UNSEEN SELF

We must keep in mind that God dwells in a secret and hidden way in all souls, in their very substance, for if He did not, they could not exist at all. This dwelling of God is very different in different souls : in some He dwells contented, in others displeased ; in some as in His own house, giving His orders and ruling it ; in others, as a stranger in a house not His own, where He is not permitted to command or to do anything at all.

(*St. John of the Cross*)

AMONG the strange experiences which have befallen me as a dream analyst none has been stranger than to witness the effect on the subject of treating seriously in the consulting-room the question : " Have I an immortal soul ? " Subjects who worked with me for a considerable time with varying improvement on the old lines laid down by the psycho-therapeutists, now tell me under treatment on the Anxiety Hypothesis, that they were aware of the importance of this before, and could not understand how it came to be overlooked. They vent their feelings of dissent at my supposed former materialism in terms which vary according to their sense of the limits of frankness. " I never began to improve really until you talked to me about the soul," says one. " I have told you this over and over again, but you took no notice," says another. Still another says : " I thought Psycho-Analysis a dreadful thing, and would have warned everybody against it, but I do not feel that about analysis of this kind." The language of another does not bear repeating.

Psychological re-education is a normative science, a science, that is to say, which lays down rules for practice. It may, therefore, be taken for granted, presumably, that the rightness of the hypothesis on which a technique is based may, in part, be estimated in terms of the practical results. Judged from this standpoint, experience goes to prove that the Anxiety Hypothesis is at least a sound *working* hypothesis, for the technique we have evolved—not perfected, by any means—at least provides a chart and compass which give us knowledge requisite for the voyage we embark upon when the problems of a new student come under discussion. This is just what a technique based on principles which have only the *biological* subject in view could not be said to yield. A case conducted on the latter lines shows no cohesion. The principles do not provide what can be called a good *working* hypothesis. It is like applying a theory of painting which teaches faithfully about brushes and colour, but not how to paint a picture. The analyst never knows where he is; unexpected developments are the rule, not the exception; an improvement, for instance, will occur unexpectedly, and a relapse come in the same way. The only thing that seems to hold the case together is the transference, and the transference elicited by the application of Freudian principles is not always of the most commendable nature. I presume that the subject is dimly aware that the process has a disintegrating effect on him, and dare not let go the one fixed point in his scheme, the analyst fulfilling in respect to the subject's psychic determinants the function of magnet.

The practical assistance provided by a method based on principles which have only the *cultural* subject in view, is scarcely less uncertain. In the absence of a use for the deeper meanings of the psycho-neurosis, recourse is had to the present-day meaning of the dream mainly, and this only touches the sphere of the stimulus, not the infantile material, *which it is the very purpose of the stimulus to awaken.*

Experience leaves no doubt, in my opinion, that the deepest concern of the psyche is directed to the question of a life *after the resolution of conflict,* and this is projected as the expectation of life after death, for, generally speaking, the resolution of the Dream-drama synchronises with death. The cycle may be recurrent, but there is no resolution expected until the fatal hour strikes for which the clock has been set at some quite early period—possibly with no date or age fixed, but the event related to some special other event in the subject's history, as, for instance, the decease of parents or of other relatives.

Religion may be regarded as a major, if not the major, projection of Anxiety. Originally, the group was the " subject." Religion gave relief from the burden of anxiety in times of danger and strain. A religion must always include two rituals, one providing a similitude of death, the other, one in which the partaking of food figures.   The first delivers from what Paul calls " this body of death," *i.e.*, the lower nature, so releasing the higher self; the second recurrently renews and builds up the higher or inner self.   Beginning with cruel initiation rites and cannibalistic feasts, these twin ideas have passed through various phases, culminating in Christianity, in Baptism, and Holy Communion. Baptism provides the similitude of death and re- birth, for which immersion in water is frequently a dream image; in Holy Communion the worshipper partakes of the Body and Blood, *i.e.*, the Soul and Life-Principle of the great Teacher and Founder.

To speak generally, the history of religion is the history of the development of the sense of sin. " The soul which sinneth, it shall die," is the original law.   But the efficacy of substitutionary sacrifices figures largely in the revelations of the Divine Purpose to the Hebrew patriarchs.   God is represented as refusing Cain's bloodless sacrifices, but as accepting Abel's slaughtered firstlings—for " without shedding of blood is no remission of sins."   Directions regarding sacrifice are a con- stant feature in the history of Abraham and his descendants.   As human life becomes more valued, the race seems vaguely restless lest animal victims should not be a sufficient substitute.   The story of Abraham's intended sacrifice of Isaac, and that of Iphigenia at Aulis, testify to this uneasiness. Human sacrifice and the sacrifice of animal victims seem to compete for precedence; holocausts of slaves, children thrown upon the glowing arms of Moloch, alternate with colossal slaughter of beasts.

Substitutionary sacrifice is the great feature of the *First Covenant*.

As the sense of sin grows heavier, and becomes individual and endopsychic, the efficacy of substitutionary sacrifice dwindles. The basis for a new covenant must be found. This new basis is provided by the teaching of Jesus. Jesus reveals the mystical life of the unseen self : the parallelism of psychology with physiology—the facts of introjection (" Not that which goeth into a man defileth a man ")—the dangers of uncontrolled projection (" but that which cometh out of a man, that defileth a man ")—the terrible fact of psychic determinism (" Unto him that hath shall be given, but from him that hath not shall be taken away even that which he hath ")—the efficacy of the immanent or indwelling God-Principle expressing itself through love and faith (miracles of healing)—above all, the mystery of re-birth.

Re-birth is the great feature of the *Second Covenant*.

All this is found again in the Anxiety Drama, as presented by the dream, the re-birth *motif* belonging particularly to the culminating phases of the drama, where the power-subject takes on himself the form of that oldest servant, woman, and rehearses in the self the supreme mystery of life won through self-surrender. But the idea of death is so integral a part of the sexuality symbol, and suffering and death are so intimately associated with sin, that the older ideas of the substitutionary sacrifice and of the inevitability of punishment spring up spontaneously along the path of every psychic storm, whether expressed in mental or physical disease.

The mechanism by which disease replaces as a symbol the parturition function is probably something like this: An organ of the body is reserved (possibly through sheer association in the infantile experience), for the seat of a mystic sacrifice. It requires to be a bodily organ presumably on the analogy of the womb; the symbol which must be at once an expiation and a similitude of birth naturally gravitates to the body. Everything else appears, from the dreams of the mental sufferer, to be counterfeit, a suggestion from the revolt subject, a machination of the subtlety of the serpent or knowledge-man. Insanity, adolescent wasting, suicide and crime may be shown to be either despair in face of the inevitable issue, or desperate attempts to evade it. When once accepted by the dream subject, the sacrifice brings not only relief, but positive joy, as I have already shown in Part II, Chapter 4. The reserved site of the expiatory suffering is especially sacred—it suggests the dream figure of a sanctuary where God meets His worshippers, and frequently the consecrated organ is referred to in the dream actually under the symbol of altar, church or temple; the service is the suffering. Or, in the extreme picture of surrender, the body may be the cross on which is hung, as expiatory offering, the self. It is a picture of surrender which baffles the

imagination of the average man; it compels his
wonder and reverence; it transcends his sympathy.
Interpreting the story of Jesus in the light of
dream analysis, I venture to think that the utterances He made on the historic journey to Jerusalem,
although in all probability implying prophetic insight, do not *necessarily* mean that He anticipated
a violent death, but that He was expressing in a
mystical figure His entire surrender to the Divine
Will. If this is so, in using the simile of crucifixion, He was employing probably an old and quite
general figure of torture, a rival of the dream image
of fire which is so common in Paul. The simile of
crucifixion is found used practically identically in
Plato's " Republic." We have noticed[1] that the
little boy of 2 years and 10 months of age represents
the human figure (Jesus, he calls it), by what to the
astonished teacher resembles a cross. It may be
that it is the cross which, in the first instance, promotes the realistic study of the human figure—the
rival of the distorted infantile representations of
man's body, perpetuated in cartoons, in which the
abdomen is not represented at all.

The history of religion and the study of dream
analysis, in fine, both demonstrate the fact that in
the very machinery of his mental life man is striving perseveringly towards one goal—reunion with
the unseen source of his being. In the course of
evolution, the sense of sin becoming more and more
endopsychic, the individual more and more turns
his regard *within* to find a mysterious sanctuary, a

[1] Page 110.

building where God may dwell with him. In the very fact of the sparking of self-consciousness, psychic material charged with affects of opposite quality is introjected, inaugurating a conflict which subserves the spiritual interests, and provides the germ of active sympathy and idealistic craving. By various devices, some of which are discussed in a former chapter, the revolt subject, *alias* the serpent or knowledge-man, labours to bring about either the commutation or the postponement of the sentence, or the transference of the punishment. He goes further than this; he endeavours, it may be, to bring a bloodless offering, some object of beauty which his own hands have wrought or his own " merit " purchased. In this connection may be quoted the following beautiful dream :—

Somebody was giving me a candlestick for a present, and I went into a shop to buy it. C. came forward to serve me. I asked to see some candlesticks; C. got on to a chair, reached down a candlestick from a glass shelf high up in the left-hand window, put a candle into it (propping it firm with a match, which annoyed me), and said it was 29s. 6d. It seemed the only one they had, and I thought it frightfully dear, but C. said it was Royal Doulton, and certainly it was very beautiful—more like a cup than a candlestick, with crimson roses on it. At this point I became aware that Mother was there too ; and C. told us that at the end of the week she was leaving the shop, and going to learn all about pottery, including designing. I said: Oh, I wish I could do that. I should love to learn designing," seeing as I spoke a vision of my own hands moulding clay to my own designs. But I knew that for some reason the training was impossible for me. I wanted it so badly that my eyes were full of hot tears and my throat ached, and I turned away, pretending to look at other things in the shop, so that Mother and C. shouldn't see me crying.

Commenting on this dream, the subject says :

In "the candlestick dream," when C. said she was leaving the shop and going to learn all about pottery, including designing, I felt an overwhelming desire (which haunted me for many subsequent days and nights) to go and do likewise. I had a sudden vision of a whirling potter's wheel, and of wet clay, with my hands moulding it to my own designs, and I longed passionately to translate the vision into actuality. The pottery in the shop was so lovely in colour and shape and texture. I *ached* with desire to produce similar works, not shrinking from the pain and effort needful before shapeless unbeautiful lumps of clay could be transformed into perfect vessels; but I wanted them to be *mine*—something actually born of me, and expressing me. If it was only the Power Subject's desire to mould life, there was yet an intense wish that my handiwork should be good and beautiful, and of service. And it came to me, in meditating on the dream, that my deep-seated wish for death, as the gateway into wider life, was, after all, merely the thwarted Power Subject's desire to have no more of anything that will not conform to his wishes. I wanted to end a

life that seemed to hold nothing further that was
worth while, and to enter into Life more abundant.
Omar Khayyam says it exactly :—

> Ah, Love, couldst thou and I with Fate conspire
> To grasp this sorry Scheme of Things entire,
>   Would we not shatter it to bits—and then
> Remould it nearer to the Heart's Desire ?

In a satisfactory dream analysis the subjective
revelations appear to follow a course proceeding in
the main line backwards from the present-day experience into remoter and more infantile experience.
The following dream, therefore, which had presented itself before the one about the beautiful
candlestick, would refer to a later psychological
situation, one in which the pessimism of the candlestick dream is yielding to an attitude more receptive
in respect to the expiatory phase. The subject had
a severe physical condition, treated three times by
surgical operation, which had moved her to seek
psychological re-education :—

*I was having tea on a gravelled terrace outside a
house, with one other woman. There was a
diamond-shaped flower bed, edged with box, close
to my feet. A man selling flowers came, but we
refused to buy. As he went away, something hurt
or sad in his appearance touched us, and we decided
to buy all he had. I ran after him, and brought
him back. He put his basket down on to the
ground, and then we saw that he had only violets
and wild rose berries, all dead. The berries were*

bruised and devoid of leaves, and the violets, dis-
coloured and limp, gave out a dreadful dead scent.
There was " no beauty, that we should desire
them," but having said that we would buy them all,
there was no going back.

It will now be in place to indicate some of the
symbols which may be taken as belonging to a category to which is appropriate the name of soul, as
that word is popularly used. The following list
does not exhaust the number.

In several places in this little book, as well as in
the *Psychology of Self Consciousness,* the *child*
has been spoken of as the supreme symbol of
the re-born self. The marital act and its natural
consequence, the new life, present the complete picture of surrender and re-birth, but this symbolism,
of course, belongs at earliest to the adolescent phase.
Prior to this the idea that there is something which
will survive the cataclysm of nature, something en-
during which neither flood nor fire destroys, persistently haunts dreams which are apparently quite
infantile. Before the sexuality symbol can have
any precise meaning for the waking consciousness,
those substances in the body which have superior
durability embody the idea of the soul. Their
presence is the first indication of the reaching out
of the mind after an unseen self which is incorrup-
tible. Stories about the hair growing after death,
of teeth surviving destruction by fire, and of the
skeleton remaining intact after disintegration of the
softer tissues, appeal to the child's imagination.

These objects are therefore chosen to represent the soul *on the principle of superior durability*. To have a tooth extracted was long ago recognised as equivalent in the dream symbolism to giving birth to a child. These two things are equivalents because both tooth and child represent something which survives the " parent "[1] body; also, to have a tooth extracted and to give birth to a child are situations which at different stages carry the suggestion of supreme suffering. To the little child tooth extraction can therefore stand as the symbol of the death into life for which, at a later stage, childbirth is the standard image. The symbolism of hair is one of the most difficult of dream problems. Hair figures prominently in the dreams of women, probably because hair-brushing and hair-cutting are more dreaded by children than is generally supposed. Also, the hair is regarded, especially in the case of girls, as a thing of beauty, and one which must, at all costs, be kept clean and in order. It is the " crown of glory " for some dreamers. Nail-cutting and nail-cleansing, also, would seem to entail more suffering than later experience alone would warrant us in assuming. A dream quoted elsewhere of the devil cutting the nails shows this aspect of the process very strongly.

Another class of soul symbols shows that the child's imagination is impressed by the fact that certain animals are *at home in a medium to which the child is a stranger*. These are notably the fish and the bird. The fish is a lowly kind of creature;

[1] Parent= bringing forth.

nevertheless, it is a persistent dream image to which a sacrosanct significance attaches. The following dream presents an admirable example of this : " *I notice a boy who has a fish in a jar in which there is not enough water. I am angry, take the boy by the scruff of the neck and insist that he shall get more water to put into the jar. I hope that someone who is with me will notice my solicitude about the fish.*" The jar is the thoracic cavity, and the dream associations include appropriately fears of pleurisy. In infantile soul symbols the power aspect of the Life Principle may be said to be more prominent than the complementary aspect of expiation.

As the child is so helpless this greater emphasis on power preserves the balance for him.

Associated with the above dream of the fish in the jar is one in which a parrot is the soul symbol. The parrot is a wise and knowing creature, inspiring fear. In the dream the *subject teases it, when it becomes almost vicious, the head getting larger and larger and appearing finally to wear a mask. In fear, the dreamer throws a tablecloth over the bird, and escapes from the room.* The bodily complaint mentioned in associations which is to reduce the fearsome soul symbol, is indigestion. The dream associations go back to a shock which the subject received as a little boy, through a practical joke in which a lighted-up mask played a part. The lad was so terrified that he had to be forcibly restrained from flinging himself down the well of the staircase.

Birds probably always carry in some way the suggestion of a higher self. The bird seems a much more fitting emblem than the fish of the higher as-

pect of the unseen life.   Dreams about birds are
very common and extremely various.   It must
be remembered that the fact of possessing a
soul may not always appear an unmitigated blessing to the juvenile subject.   As the Life-Principle
may assume even the aspect of devil when in its
directive function it elicits hate, so the soul may
masquerade as a vicious old parrot when the sacrifices entailed on its behalf are not appreciated.[1]   The
bird lends itself to every aspect under which the soul
principle can be conceived, from the gentle dove
which carries the olive branch over the waste of
waters, to the bird of prey which anticipates that
the less honourable parts of the self shall provide
it with a carrion meal.   The child's attitude to the
call of suffering will be the deciding factor when the
choice of the symbol is under consideration.   If it
is true that a God-Principle within ultimately
creates man in His own image, it is equally true,
from the dream, that man creates God and the soul
in images of his own invention.

The *aesthetic object* is not always associated with
the revolt in quite the same way as it is in the dream
of the beautiful candlestick, given above.   On the
contrary, in most contexts, objects of artistry :
paintings, carvings, needlework, represent the
pathological bodily condition which is the seat of

[1] The same principle may account for the genesis of the witch.
In all my experience I have so far heard only one dream in which
a witch figures.   The subject was put under a spell by this witch,
and the incident involved a bottle containing ammonia.   The
dream associations go back to a self-righteous and exacting
grandmother.

expiation, and when so used they are the equivalent of the altar or church, and suggest the price paid for the soul. A subject, for instance, already quoted, dreams that *she is to take part in a bazaar. She arrives before the bazaar is formally opened, and is looking over the objects which are to be sold. The one she notices is a dressing-table cover, worked in cross-stitch.* This article is a typical dream image for the bodily condition which is the expiation venture for her inner life. It is handiwork; it is beautiful; it is worked in *cross-stitch.* It is to be sold, given, *i.e.,* for standard value, and, what is more, in this particular case, it is to be sold at a bazaar, not, therefore, for immediate personal gain, but for a disinterested, possibly a religious, object. The beautiful aesthetic object which must be cherished, almost adored, is a peculiarly interesting dream image. It is generally an object which has capacity, *i.e.,* it is a receptacle, and the meaning of this may be that it is analogous to the uterus. Herein may lie the difference between the correct soul symbol and the symbol of the revolt subject (*cf.* the candlestick mentioned above). The following two dreams, both dreamed by the same subject, exemplify this double treatment of the symbol. In the first, the soul symbol is a basket, in the second, a beautiful vase. In the first the dreamer imagines herself *coming into a house, but she does not know why she has come. She is carrying a blue and silver basket made of raffia, which someone criticises severely.* The associations go to a little raffia mat which the subject made as a little child in the kin-

dergarten, to give to her mother on the occasion of
the latter's silver wedding day.   In connection with
the criticising of the basket an aunt was mentioned,
who had often criticised the subject when she was a
child.   In the second dream (not of the same day),
the dreamer saw a *very beautiful vase, the flowers
in which were faded.*   The silver and blue raffia
basket and the beautiful vase seem to represent an
inner self ; each is the special feature of the dream in
which it occurs.

I have already, in a previous chapter, commented
upon the fact that Professor Freud, overlooking, as
he does, the conflict in the genuine Unconscious,
does scant justice to the psychic conflicts of early
life.   The dreams of children are far from being
wish-fulfilments in Professor Freud's meaning of
the term.   In face of the records of night terrors
and sleep walking which are a commonplace in the
history of so many subjects in early life, such a
judgment seems remarkable.   Children sometimes
cannot be induced even to relate their dreams, on
account of the fear inspired.   Possibly, the mental
and physical well-being of the child is more often
in the balance than is supposed.   The stress of
domestication may be terrific in the case of high-
spirited children to whom the meticulous habits of
their elders are utterly incomprehensible.   Why,
asks a little girl, is a room " tidy " when the
articles in it are disposed in one particular order,
and " untidy " when disposed in any other
order ?   Some of the most capable people I have
known have told me of the utter inadequacy they

M

have felt as little children, when confronted with the task of learning quite simple accomplishments. One was perfectly certain that she would never learn to read, another that she would never be able to thread a needle. That the freedom of his own body is forgone by the child, and the disposal of his activities by others endured, only with inexpressible suffering, we may suppose; the urgency of the Problem of Suffering, so universal in some form, and in some cases so pressing, reflects in all likelihood the attitude of the adult to the problem of his own discarded infantile liberty. It has been retrospectively objectified, according to the habit of the dream-subject, and projected, probably, through association, on to some special class of beings.

I may mention, in passing, that the difficulties of adolescence appear to be scarcely less. Here the supreme symbol of the soul emerges—the child. A dream of a very large mother and a very small baby reflects with pathetic irony this bitter conflict—the expiation so great, the achievement so small! The self-criticism of this dream is remarkable, but far from uncommon.

Speaking generally, it is not only the conflict of the infantile period which is imperfectly appreciated, but the anxiety problem in general. The opinion prevails in some circles that all nervous symptoms are malingering; in others that they are signs of an inferior psychic endowment. They are stigmatised either as attempts which the weakling subject makes to get away from the tedious duties of social membership, or as compensations for the boredom, dreariness and repressions of ordinary life. The psycho-neurotic is called " selfish," he is said to " imagine " his troubles, and to take refuge in dreaming, hallucinations and phantasies, because he is too indolent or too cowardly to secure the tangible pleasures of life for himself.

Not at all! Such judgments are entirely inadequate. The problems of childhood are most indifferently understood and altogether under-rated. The bulk of sufferers are often the most sincere, the most directly moral, the least self-pleasing among mankind. There is an important distinction to be made, however. There is one class of psychic phenomena which, while most practically useful, if of a certain kind and degree, may induce self-indulgence and work the most disastrous effects. This is the waking phantasy normally arising in adolescence.

In the *Psychology of Self-Consciousness*, I have suggested a theory for the origin of such phantasies. I am under the impression that in adolescence the maturing of the sexual organs brings along with it a fresh tide of power, which is balanced by the revival of terror situations. The blend produces what is pleasurable to consciousness, and undergoes a certain amount of elaboration. The phantasy habit, functioning serviceably, performs the task of *scavenger* in respect to the buried terrors of the infantile period. These terrors it brings into contact with the animal passions associated with the reproductive function. The terrors

and the appetitive passions, now in contact, under-
go a process—shall we say of fermentation?—in
the laboratory of the subject's psychology, and, as
a result, the balance is re-established and fresh
energy thrown into the life of adulthood, the phantasy being projected as actual activities in the waking life. But too often this happy result does not follow. The phantasy-life, functioning wrongly,
fosters seductive self-indulgence and leads to
sadism, masochism and narcissism. On account
of the sexuality element in the power scale of the
balance, the waking phantasy favours more particularly the romance presentation. Hence it is the
breeding-ground of sentimentalism and porno-
graphical interest. It feeds the everyday passion
life of mankind; it floods the book-shops with indifferent or demoralising literature, and the stage
with dramatic representations of the same class. It
fosters, along with sentimentalism and undesirable
curiosity, their negative counterparts, hate and
jealousy, projected against persons of the environment, although in reality directed against the self.
The " ruling passion " takes its rise in the phantasy life, whether for good or for bad. It is the
waking phantasy, functioning uncontrolled, which
arouses, in the hard-headed, misgivings as to the
genuine usefulness of cultivating the interests—at
any rate, any beyond those of ordinary religion—
of the inner life. A doubt is cast for these people
on the seriousness of all human purpose which is
not immediately practical. They shun the theatre,
and the library where works of the imagination are

to be found. But to think of the imagination as if it were merely a mechanism for securing seductive indulgence is really a monstrous calumny of human nature, and leads to starvation of the inner interests. The burden of this is felt by the poets, and it has moved many to undertake an apology of their art. Among moderns, Shelley has done this.[1] In his *apologia*, the poet is protesting against the opprobrium which attaches in the mind of the practical or narrowly God-fearing man to this highest faculty of human nature.

The conscious phantasy habit is part of the faculty which we know as the *Imagination; it is the least part.* In deeper recesses of the psycho-physical sphere the imagination works the miracle which we know as MAN. In its mirror, the physical experiences of life are wrought into something new and higher, leaving, it may be, the waking life, relatively cold. This coldness Carlyle refers to as the " Centre of Indifference through which whoso travels from the Negative Pole to the Positive Pole must necessarily pass."

The Centre of Indifference is the state in which emotion working from deeper levels leaves the waking consciousness a free field for the exercise of judgment.

Whereas excessive phantasy decentralises energy, robbing the inner life, by bringing symbolic efficacy into the physical in undue amount, the proper exercise of the imagination throws back animal energy into the spiritual for transmutation. To

[1] See Appendix I, No. 2.

indulge phantasy unlawfully is to have your treasure on earth, to transmute lower into spiritual energy is to have your treasure in heaven.[1]

The dream must always be distinguished from the waking phantasy, *the genuine dream being wholly serious in purpose.* How far the dream embodies the waking phantasy is an important question. I am under the impression that the dream itself ridicules the phantasy life, or at least that part of it which disturbs its own serious purpose, by importing fragments of phantasy into the dream as images of a very diminutive size and by other mechanisms.

The dream life holds the key of what we call the conscience. It expresses the ethical conflict in man; it is a source of willing. We fear the dream life, and therefore disregard it. It is too serious in the hour of joy, too awful or too painful in the hour of collapse. But dislocation between the two levels of consciousness is the root of all disaster, and therefore the dream compels attention.

[1] In an Illustrative Exercise on the *Pied Piper* an Associate of the Psychological Aid Society describes the psychology of the phantasy habit. (See Appendix II.)

CONCLUSION

THE human mind has from time immemorial been haunted by the idea that life here is complemented by existence of another kind. Indeed, belief in existence after death may be said to be the most characteristic and fundamental of all human cravings. It is the slender bond which unites the most divergent races, and the most divergent individuals of any given race. It is in the mind of the little Eastern woman who claps her hands and rings a bell at the wayside shrine to attract the attention of the Dweller within; and equally it is in the mind of Monsignor, as he assists at High Mass in a prosaic European capital. At every turn in the road the serpent, or knowledge-man, awaits the unwary, and asks: " *Is* this thing true; *hath* God said? " And the man who does not immediately repel these insinuations and turn a deaf ear to the charmer will, whether he knows it or not, probably have cause to rue the trafficking with his own unbelief before the sands of his hour-glass have run out. Nietzsche is a great warning. Is our insistent belief in an afterlife a superstition which we have to outgrow?—or is it a part of the eternal constitution of that Great Unknowable which we call Life, to the understanding of which all our conquests in science may bring us nearer if the revolt subject in us is only treated with straightforward honesty, and turned into an ally instead of being allowed to remain a hidden enemy or a dreaded adversary? The young man who, when his own dreams were being discussed with him on Freudian principles, exclaimed: " Is the world, then, not rational? " was voicing something quite stupendous. At the time I asked myself anxiously what he could mean; but as I had only undertaken psychology to do, as I put it, donkey work for my medical friends, I suspended judgment and awaited results.

Further research has led me to different conclusions from those entertained by all the psychotherapists among my medical friends, except one, and I am bound to say that the evidence of the dream life is all in favour of life having just the rationality of which that subject was thinking, how far consciously I do not know.[1] The testimony of mankind in waking consciousness is not without a witness in the deepest place in the human heart. I now realise that to associate dreaming with a call to a higher life is the only adequate interpretation of the Ego-urge. It is because the two classes of reality, the spiritual and the material, become dislocated, that the human economy suffers as it does. The more sensitive and cultivated the race becomes, the more it must break down, in body or mind, or both, unless it can devise a plan for getting both classes of reality into one sweep of vision—unless, indeed, it learns, as said before, to have what Jesus calls " the single eye."

Through Christian Science and Spiritual Heal-

---

[1] See above page 139, and also below page 178.

ing, the race is endeavouring to do this thing empirically. Is there not a Science and Art which will promote it? Is there not a type of psychological educator who will step into the breach? I mistrust the doctor, *qua* doctor, not the individual, but the traditions of the profession. Is not the emblem of this art just that serpent who is the ancient enemy of mankind? Paracelsus expressed this mistrust of the medical profession in the Middle Ages, and Sir Thomas Browne did no less. It is the strangest irony which has made a profession, whose emblem is the serpent, the masters of mankind. Besides, the functions of physician and psychologist, as the words imply, are separate, and both are needed.

Why hide our ignorance under an assumption of learning? Let us cultivate the meekness of wisdom. Paranoia is marked by the extreme of positive affirmation. Let us say frankly when we do not know, and not encourage *a will for certainty at all costs*. Frankly, *we do not know* what life is; we do not know what psychic phenomena are, multiple personalities, hallucinations, phantasms. To describe is not to explain. To confound description and explanation is a gross error, one all too common in these days of " quick returns." To explain *relations*, as science aims at doing, is to come a step nearer, but never do we reach the final *nexus*, and with Kant, we must assume God, *i.e.*, a universal Life concept, behind a double series of experience, a subjective series and an objective series. This is not *a* way, it is *the* way.

It is *the way of the dream life*, and experience

proves that if the dream life is out of gear the whole man is affected in his development in some direction. The mind of man refuses to believe that this elaborate and rational scheme of things, which we call the Universe or Cosmos, and which more and more we learn to know through the medium of science, breaks down in respect to man, the culminating revelation. The feeling is that human survival is the only adequate interpretation for the immense life-urge which man feels. Does the Life-Principle create appetitions for which it has no satisfaction? We cannot, of course, know the answer to this by quite the same line of research that we know the answer to many things, but when man has sufficiently purged his mind of infantile fears he may discover methods of research in these fields which will fulfil all the conditions of logic. As I see the problem in the consulting room, I realise that more and more mankind tends to become sick in mind and body—or, failing this, wicked, if only selfish and bad-tempered—because in the waking life, the diffusion of knowledge has thrown, for an increasing number of people, doubts on the question of human survival, and in the deep psyche the life-urge in this direction is so strong that it will not be gainsaid. It cries out all the louder the more we try to drown it in the waking life. Doubt of survival strikes at the root of human purpose, at the root of the sense of responsibility, and at the root of the otherwise unquenchable idealism and self-sacrifice of the human soul. It also strikes at the root of physical health.

When we look critically at the re-education process, a physiological factor appears to associate itself with the demand. I realise that in the course of a dream analysis, something happens to what we may call the Life Energy of the subject. As he first presents himself, the obviously pathological subject appears to be guarding something—brooding over something from which he fears to have his attention distracted. In time, the nature of this discloses itself. It is reserve energy of some sort. The principles of the pioneers in dream analysis encourage the abreaction, *i.e.,* setting loose, of this displaced energy which may be the *dirt* of the dream symbolism. Abreaction is decentralisation, and very often there results from mere abreaction a certain release of tension which has the appearance of giving relief. But in a fairly large proportion of cases I observe that the relief, if it follows, is one-sided. If the mental symptoms are relieved there may be other undesirable results to balance the advantage ; somatic ones, for instance. The see-saw action between mind and body attracted my attention more than it did that of my medical colleagues, who were accustomed to think of mental states together with functional disorders, as belonging to an entirely different category from organic diseases. Experience convinces me more and more that this distinction is drawn too rigorously.

There is a mysterious dream image, the " plate," associated with the problem I am discussing. This plate must probably be taken in the sense of *clamp* (*cf.* " plate-laying " in railway construction), but it also covers other ideas, which are duly provided for by the symbolism of the dinner plate.[1] This plate could, I suppose, symbolise a synapse, conceivably. In conjunction with this problem, also, there is generally a great deal said about the storeys of a house, especially in connection with going up and down stairs. The correlation of these dream symbols with different levels of the nervous system is too pointed to be overlooked.

What is it that the subject fears? What is he watching? Why does he dread to be distracted from his watch? To theorise rather adventurously, I may suggest that the situation would be explained if we could assume that two charges of some energy like electricity, of opposite signs, were threatening to discharge themselves and re-combine in the somatic sphere. The subject will often go to any lengths of resistance, including lapses into insanity, in order to prevent this. If we could imagine the two aspects of the Life-force, Power and Expiation, as charges of energy of opposite signs, and take the body as the " earth," we should have a complete picture of the process on the analogy of two charges of electricity becoming " earthed." For the complete rehabilitation of the subject, the method, it seems, is to interpret the dream in terms of a symbolism which brings the spiritual life into prominence. This may sound mystical, but it works. *Somewhere in a super-physical sphere, apparently,*

[1] In science the word " plate " is not overlooked in connection with the nervous system.

the opposite charges may spark safely. The pressure is great, but the " transference " supports the subject during the process. In extreme cases, perhaps, the " transference " involves the delegation, *pro tem.*, to the re-educator of the waking directive function. Strictly speaking, wherever possible, the transference should not involve a delegation of authority, but be a co-partnership, and such a co-partnership will in due time result, if the re-educator can exercise patience, and avail himself of opportunities.[1]

The process of the dream work, when the dream is interpreted on the lines of the Anxiety Hypothesis, may be described as *transmuting* energy. The more intense emotion vanishes, relegated, presumably, into some sphere where the interests of the inner unseen self are the business in hand. All concern of the psyche is seen to attach ultimately to these interests. At any rate, the subject's difficulties are more easily and naturally susceptible of control through re-education on these lines than on any other, I find. When this method is employed, the reserved energy appears to rise in the nervous system to higher levels.

The energy in question in the discussion of these problems appears to be nothing which the physiologist can investigate. The only term at all applicable to it is Life-energy. *Many dream symbols represent it.* Experiments on food-stuffs and organic tissues are simply irrelevant in connection

[1] In my experience the re-educator needs three essential qualities—courage, the meekness of wisdom and infinite love.

with it, and experiments described by psycho-physiologists on the gross results of emotional disturbances in animals, caused by graduated fear and other stimuli, with or without the removal of glandular tissue, do not touch the central problem, which is that of human endopsychic autonomy. The psyche in the dream is her own judge, her own advocate, her own prosecutor, her own executioner, in respect to all elements introjected in the period of life which sees the rise of conceptual thought processes. The thing of chief importance in the unearthing of the conflict is to treat it as the really remote thing that it is, as a drama which is being enacted not on one stage (or screen) alone—the dream—but which is apt also to be reflected (or projected) on to the bodily organs and tissues, and on to the subject's reactions to life. This separation of experience will help forward to a unification of the economy which makes for health and sanity.

Why did the young man employ the word *rational* in conjunction with the latent content of dreams?[1] Probably he could not altogether have justified his use of the term, but the fact that he did so use it suggests some interesting speculations. *Rational* does not seem on the first encounter an appropriate term, but a deeper knowledge of the infantile psychology in reference to the surrender of animal preoccupations in favour of conceptual ones may show that it is not out of place. There appears to be a deep down sense that in connection with the surrender there are expectations of a *quid pro quo*.

[1] See above, pages 139 and 172.

In consciousness many subjects express a willingness that death shall be extinction, but in the unconscious I doubt whether there is the same unconcern. In the organic or perceptual realm *do ut des* (I give that you may in your turn give) may be good enough for waking consciousness; but it is not good enough in the dawning conceptual. Here, the anguish of the surrender is real—a mutilated animal, a butcher's shop, are symbols befitting its intensity. Salvation is conceived as bought, bought with a price; lapses are paid for, and dearly paid for; but always the subject expects that faith will be kept with him, and that some reward awaits him. If the term *rational* is in place here, then *rational,* in the first instance, means *faithful to a covenant,* and is a synonym for righteous.

So urgent is the matter for the dream consciousness that a discrediting, in the waking consciousness, of the scheme of salvation brings with it a dislocation of the two levels which results ultimately in some kind of breakdown.

The idea is supported by negative, as well as by positive, evidence. A subject, for instance, with a great deal of mental disturbance, after a course of Freudian study, dreamed that he *passed by* on a higher road a scene in which a goat was being put to death. The directive personality, preoccupied with the study of the biological subject in himself in waking consciousness, is here shown as estranged from the expiation process which has been neglected. The dream indicates the danger of dissociation in cases of obstinate infantile opposi-

tion, or indifference, to the strict ethical code of the
dream life; a counterpart picture to the normal attitude to salvation is then presented. In these cases
the expectation in the dream that the reward will
follow is replaced by a fear that it will be forfeited.
When the casket shall be opened, which should
contain the precious jewel of immortality, there will
be NOTHING. The subject is, in his own eyes,
beyond hope. He is, if not the suicide, one who
presents the picture of despair or incapacity. Short
of this Faustus transaction, the subject *expects*
redemption.   His sufferings may be great, but he
confidently anticipates that he will see of the
travail of his soul, and will be satisfied.

So much stress has been laid on the unseen aspect
of experience in the preceding pages that the en-
quirer may, perhaps, ask what function remains for
the waking consciousness.   It is impossible to do
anything like justice to this aspect of the enquiry,
but a few words may be in place in concluding.

Conceptual experience in waking consciousness
must be valued as being of the first importance. To
it belong the projection of the Self concept, and the
objective shaping of the character in a group.   Life
on the material plane constitutes, we may believe,
a highly valuable part of the psyche's training.

In *The Psychology of Self-Consciousness*, I
have likened the manifestations of the Life-
Principle on this globe to experiments on the dis-
persion of light.   As by passing through a prism,
light is broken up into its constituent parts, so by

the exigencies of phenomenal experience life is
distributed in such a way as to present an emotional
spectrum. Again, as the second prism recombines
the rays of light, so for the conceptual subject tradition and re-education restore unity to the character,
a unity enriched, we may believe, by the fact of the
distributing process. We may with Browning
cry :

" All good things are ours, nor soul helps flesh
more now, than flesh helps soul ! "

Dream analysis shows that within limits it is not
the *quality of experience* that matters, but the *fact
of experience,* together with the insight of the subject as regards his own problem.

Phenomenal experience, like boarding-school, is
a period of training away from the intimacies of
home among others who are at once peers and com-
petitors. In such an environment the inner unity
of Selfhood is confirmed, and at the same time the
emergent aspects of character acquire a solidarity
and a certain sharpness of definition.

The soteriological schemes of the unconscious
psyche, are, by projection, put to the test of service-
ability to group life, and experience shows that
some must be eliminated in the interests of fellow-
group members. An example is the male tendency
to transfer expiation. This must be checked, partly
because its projection provides the Don Juan, the
defamer of character, and perhaps even the murderer, and also partly because it is not clearly to be

N

differentiated from a negative attitude to the female principle (expiation). Within reasonable limits, the transference of expiation is the mechanism of the noblest in human nature, the vehicle of compassion.

There is always a compensatory action at work in vital processes, and we find that in proportion to the magnitude of the charges of the two determinants in the " sparking," so will be the opportunities of the subject. If the introjection of more intense emotional experience releases a larger amount of negative affect (fear or hate), the amount of positive affect (love) available must be equally great. The conflict is the more intense, but the resultant unity will be proportionately valuable. Our concern must be to carry forward the unifying process, and not to let the vital energy be lost in indiscriminate projection. We must not follow the instinctive bent, which is to keep the love affects for the Self and project the negative ones, but study rather to do the opposite, to follow the *spiritual* law. This has been the high teaching of all the world's greatest, those known to fame as well as those many bright and loving spirits who have laboured among us from the first beginnings of human development, " mute," we may believe, but " inglorious," we cannot believe. They form a noble and indissoluble spiritual fraternity, and know and recognise one another across intervals of time and space; despite the barriers erected by race and class all sincere conceptual subjects are " in touch." That is why the sayings of a Lao-Tze or a Christ, of an

Epictetus or a Marcus Aurelius, of a Browning, or a Paul, *all* appeal to every reader who is of the genuine conceptual fraternity. There is not unison but there is harmony in the utterances of the great.

It has been said above that we do not understand ultimate experience, that it is indescribable—occult. We cannot convey to another person the most trifling fact of experience, whether pleasurable or painful, except in terms of common experience. The description of ultimate experience is—to use the word quite generally—mysticism.

We can only describe experience in terms of its physical accompaniments; that is why the mystic, in endeavouring to impart interior experience, employs analogy. All analogy starts from and must associate itself with the nuclear group of symbolism, which brings body and unseen self into relation, and physical pleasure and pain into relation with sorrow and joy.

The difficulties of communication are so great that for practical purposes the human psyche has tended to give up doing what has all the appearance of an impossibility, and hence arises what we call in psychology " dissociation." The facts of experience which we cannot describe or communicate are shut away from the rest of consciousness. Whenever a mental symptom, of whatever gravity, appears in the psychological life, it is a sign that the dissociated elements are too dynamic to remain in ward. The dream shows the mechanism of dissociation most plainly. For instance, a dreamer *sees a child with the private parts covered with a rash. The dream subject thinks " measles ! " and reflects that it will not do for her to let the other children and the grown-ups, of whom several are present, see the state the child is in, in case there should be a panic.* The indication is quite correct, as a severe epidemic of measles from which members of the subject's family suffered was a most significant factor in her psychological history.

It must not be admitted that mysticism is altogether outside the scope of psychology, or human science fails in the crowning and crucial test. Mark Rutherford voices this in the words :

> " Hitherto science has been mainly the subjugation of the external world. I dream sometimes of a science which shall be cultivated as physical science is now, but shall have for its object our private peace and happiness; for example the harmonising and guidance of the imagination. At present we fight naked and no better armed than our ancestors of 2,000 years ago." [1]

The Life-Principle has impregnated the material and its offspring are all organic forms. Man may explore up to a point the subjective as well as the objective aspects of these vast cosmic facts, and the dream study in the light of the Anxiety Hypothesis helps us on the way to a solution of the stupendous riddle. It informs us that the development of human knowledge in both directions—the

[1] *Last Pages of a Journal.*

subjective and the objective—is fundamentally interlocked. Without the assistance of the dream this secret has been penetrated before by schools of mystics. Modern psychology cannot afford to ignore it if it is to be of practical value to any extent. William James was alive to the importance of the subjective side. He writes: " Our normal waking consciousness is but one special type of consciousness, while all about it, parted from it by the flimsiest of screens, there lie potential forms of consciousness entirely different. We may go through life without suspecting their existence, but apply the requisite stimuli, and at a touch they are there." And again: " The further limits of our being plunge into an altogether other dimension of existence from the sensible and merely understandable world. Name it the mystical region or the supernatural region, whichever you choose."

The interesting psychological phenomenon known as "resistance" is one not unimportant piece of evidence for the fact that the dream study is akin to the mystic side of experience. Freudian dream philosophy has made us familiar with the doctrine of the resistance even when analysis is not carried below what I contend is still within the sphere of the symbolic—the human body and its functions. Resistance strengthens when the veil of symbolism is lifted, as the attitude of the Freudian psychologists itself illustrates in an illuminating fashion. The adept in mysticism is thoroughly alive to the resistance and warns the initiate in no mistakable terms against the exploration of problems for which he is at the moment unprepared spiritually. George Herbert says :

> Avoid profaneness; come not here !
> Nothing but holy, pure and clear,
> Or that which groaneth to be so,
> May at his peril farther go.[1]

[1] From *Superluminare* (The Threshold)

APPENDIX I

1. THE LAW IS WITHIN. Extract from Voltaire.

2. THE RESPECTIVE FUNCTIONS OF THE REASON AND THE IMAGINATION. Extract from *A Defence of Poetry*, by Shelley.

3. THE OFFICE OF FRIENDSHIP. Extracts from (a) Dante's *Paradise*, canto II; (b) *Essay on Love*, by Emerson.

4. RE-ABSORPTION OF NEGATIVE INTO THE SELF. Extract from James Hinton.

5. THE UNIVERSAL LAW OF BALANCE. Extracts from the *Essay on Compensation*, by Emerson, and the introductory poem attached to the Essay.

6. SURRENDER ASPECT OF THE LIFE PRINCIPLE AT THE LEVEL OF THE ANIMAL KINGDOM. *Wild Flowers*, George Macdonald.

APPENDIX II

ILLUSTRATIVE EXERCISE ON *The Pied Piper*, by Miss Alison.

APPENDIX I

No. 1

The Law is Within

Si Dieu n'est pas dans nous, il n'exista jamais. . . .
Je ne puis ignorer ce qu'ordonna mon maître.
Il m'a donné sa loi, puisqu'il m'a donné l'être. . . .
La morale uniforme en tout temps, en tout lieu,
A, dès siècles sans fin, parlé au nom de ce Dieu.
C'est la loi de Trajan, de Socrate, et la vôtre,
De ce culte éternel la nature est l'apôtre.
Le bon sens le reçoit ; et les remords vengeurs,
Nés de la conscience, en sont les défenseurs.

(VOLTAIRE)

P. 5 (a).

No. 2

The Respective Functions of Reason and the Imagination

ACCORDING to one mode of regarding those two classes of mental action which are called reason and imagination, the former may be considered as mind contemplating the relations borne by one thought to another, however produced; and the latter as mind acting upon those thoughts so as to colour them with its own light and composing from them, as from elements, other thoughts, each containing within itself the principle of its own integrity. The one is the τὸ ποιεῖν or principle of synthesis, and has for its object those forms which are common to universal nature and existence itself; the other the τὸ λογίζειν or principle of analysis, and its action regards the relation of things simply as relations; considering thoughts, not in their integral unity, but as the algebraical representations which conduct to certain results. Reason is the enumeration of quantities already known; imagination is the perception of the value of those quantities both separately and as a whole. Reason respects the differences and imagination the similitudes of things. Reason is to imagination as the instrument to the agent, as the body to the spirit, as the shadow to the substance.

PERCY BYSSHE SHELLEY, *Defence of Poetry*.
Pp. 47 and 48.

No. 3

The Office of Friendship

(a)

The increate perpetual thirst that draws
Towards the realm of God's own form, bore us
Swift almost as the heaven ye behold.
Beatrice upward gazed, and I on her ;
*   *   *   *   *   *   *
Whence she, to whom no care of mine was hid,
Turning to me, with aspect glad as fair,
Bespake me : " Gratefully direct thy mind
To God, through Whom to this first star we come."
                              Dante (*Paradise*, canto II)

(b)

THERE are moments when the affections rule and
absorb the man and make his happiness dependent
on a person or persons.   But in health the mind is
presently seen again—its overarching vault, bright
with galaxies of immutable lights, and the warm
loves and fears that swept over us as clouds must
lose their finite character and blend with God, to
attain their own perfection.   But we need not fear
that we can lose anything by the progress of the
soul.   The soul may be trusted to the end.   That
which is so beautiful and attractive, as these relations, must be succeeded and supplanted only by
what is more beautiful, and so on for ever.

Essay on Love by RALPH WALDO EMERSON.

No. 4

Re-absorption of " Negative " Affects into the Self.

INTELLECTUALLY, the world is a mystery to us;
morally, a fearful problem. Am I wrong in saying
that there is a remedy for this state of things in
remembering that man's deficiency modifies his impressions and convictions and in endeavouring to
ascertain in what respect the very fact that is, must
exceed what is, to his consciousness. That is tech-
nically to find out and exclude the negative element
in his perception by taking it into himself. If we
will do that, the clouds roll back, the darkness turns
to light. Nothing is altered, but we understand.

The Mystery of Pain, by JAMES HINTON.
P. 63.

No. 5
The Universal Law of Balance

The wings of Time are black and white,
Pied with morning and with night.
Mountain tall and ocean deep
Trembling balance duly keep.
In changing moon, in tidal wave,
Glows the feud of Want and Have.

. . . .

POLARITY, or action and reaction, we meet in every part of nature, in darkness and light, in heat and cold, in the ebb and flow of waters, in male and female, in the inspiration and expiration of plants and animals, in the equation of quantity and quality, in the fluids of the animal body, in the systole and diastole of the heart, in the undulations of fluids and of sound, in the centrifugal and centripetal gravity, in electricity, galvanism and chemical affinity. Superinduce magnetism at one end of the needle, the opposite magnetism takes place at the other end. If the south attracts, the north repels. To empty here, you must condense there. An inevitable dualism bisects nature, so that each thing is half and suggests another thing to make it whole : as spirit, matter ; man, woman ; odd, even ; subjective, objective ; in, out ; upper, under ; motion, rest ; yea, nay.

While the world is thus dual, so is every one of its parts. The entire system of things gets represented in every particle. There is somewhat that resembles the ebb and flow of the sea, day and night, man and woman, in a single needle of the pine, in a kernal of corn, in each individual of every tribe. The reaction so grand in the elements is repeated within these small boundaries.

Essay on Compensation by RALPH WALDO EMERSON.
P. 64.

No. 6

Surrender Aspect of the Life Principle at the Level of the Vegetable Kingdom

Do ye know when the spoilers near you come
By a shuddering in your gloom ?
For blind and deaf we think you are,
Hearing, seeing, near nor far.
Is it so ?
Is it only ye are dumb ?
Yet alive, at least, I think,
Trembling almost on the brink
Of our lonely consciousness.
If this be so—
Take this comfort for your woe :
For the breaking of your root,
For the rending in your breast,
For the blotting of the sun,
For the death too soon begun ;
For all else beyond redress—
For the thing ye cannot be,
That the children's wonder-springs
Bubble high at sight of you.
Lovely, lowly, common things—
More blessing than they see,
When they float into their view.
That ye, bravely creeping out,
Smile away our manhood's doubt,
And our childhood's faith renew,
And that we, with old age nigh,
Seeing you alive and well,
Out of winter's crucible,
Ye who from the grave have crept,
Telling us, ye have only slept—
Think we die not, though we die,
Thus, ye die not though ye die—
Only yield your being up
Like a nectar-holding cup.
Deaf, ye give to them that hear
With a greatness, lovely, dear ;
Blind, ye give to them that see ;
Poor, yet bounteous royally—
Lowly servants to the higher,
Burning upwards on the fire
Of Nature's endless sacrifice.

P. 64.   *Wild Flowers*   GEORGE MACDONALD.

APPENDIX II

Illustrative Exercise on the Pied Piper

" THE DREAM,[1] in placing before the subject the story of the ' Pied Piper,' would have chosen the City of Hamelin to represent the subject himself. The townsfolk would represent the Soul; the Corporation, the Intellect, and the Mayor, the Will; for, as the people are the life of the city, and express themselves in it, and live in it subject to the government of the Mayor and Corporation, so the Soul is the life of the Body and lives in it, subject to the government of the Will and the Intellect.

" In this case the people of the city were made miserable by a plague which made the city unfit to live in, and they went to the Mayor and Corporation and begged them to take steps to put an end to it, blaming them for their laziness in allowing this nuisance to persist. Just so the Soul, if worried by some form of sin which may express itself in some bodily ailment, will approach the Will with the voice of conscience : the subject will suffer under his fault and blame himself for his inertia. The Mayor of the story is represented as greedy, fat, and lazy ; and, with the Corporation, he sits idly revolving the difficulty, but does not make any useful suggestion.

[1] Miss Alison's treatment of the subject is in certain respects slightly different from my own. The point is that she brings out so well the Pied Piper as the function of phantasy. She shows that, whereas up to a certain point phantasy is capable of doing the subject a service, beyond those limits and without certain precautions it may be harmful.

" The Piper himself may represent Phantasy; a means by which the evil is temporarily removed, or apparently so. He removes the rats, but he does not remove the conditions which allowed the city to get into this verminous state. Phantasy, by turning the thoughts into different channels, may remove the evil for the time being; but unless the Will and Intellect then co-operate, and the subject takes steps to discipline himself and strike at the root of the trouble, to show his goodwill towards the power which has shown him the way of deliverance and to pay for what has been done for him, his condition will be worse than it was before.

" In this case the Mayor and Corporation were not prepared to pay the price; the subject was lazy and allowed himself to get into the power of Phantasy insteady of putting himself right with it; and for this cause the children of the city, the young growing life of the soul, were taken away. The soul was warped and thrown back in its development because its interests were neglected by the Will and the Intellect. But since hope always remains, one child was left.

" The children were taken by the Piper into an underground cavern, where in time they grew up and apparently emerged in Transylvania, where they and their descendants caused much comment by their odd ways. Just so if the energy of the soul is distorted and pushed into wrong channels, it will express itself in eccentricity and abnormal behaviour, and possibly a dissociation of the personality may take place."